Lighting the
Lamp of Wisdom

Other books in the
A Week Inside Series

Lighting the Lamp of Wisdom

A Week Inside a Yoga Ashram

John Ittner

Foreword by
Dr. David Frawley (Pandit Vamadeva Shastri)

Walking Together, Finding the Way
SKYLIGHT PATHS Publishing
Woodstock, Vermont

Lighting the Lamp of Wisdom:
A Week Inside a Yoga Ashram

© 2002 by John Ittner
Foreword © 2002 by Dr. David Frawley

Library of Congress Cataloging-in-Publication Data
Ittner, John, 1951–
Lighting the lamp of wisdom : a week inside a yoga ashram / John Ittner ;
foreword by David Frawley.
          p.   cm.
Includes bibliographical references.
ISBN 1-893361-52-7 (Paperback) — ISBN 1-893361-37-3 (Hardcover)
1. Spiritual retreats—Hinduism. 2. Ashrams. 3. Yoga. I. Title.
BL1238.72 .I88 2002
294.5'65—dc21   2002010512

10 9 8 7 6 5 4 3 2 1

Manufactured in the United States of America

SkyLight Paths Publishing is creating a place where people of different spiritual traditions come together for challenge and inspiration, a place where we can help each other understand the mystery that lies at the heart of our existence.

SkyLight Paths sees both believers and seekers as a community that increasing-ly transcends traditional boundaries of religion and denomination—people wanting to learn from each other, *walking together, finding the way.*

SkyLight Paths, "Walking Together, Finding the Way" and colophon are trademarks of LongHill Partners, Inc., registered in the U.S. Patent and Trademark Office.

Walking Together, Finding the Way
Published by SkyLight Paths Publishing
A Division of LongHill Partners, Inc.
Sunset Farm Offices, Route 4, P.O. Box 237
Woodstock, VT 05091
Tel: (802) 457-4000 Fax: (802) 457-4004
www.skylightpaths.com

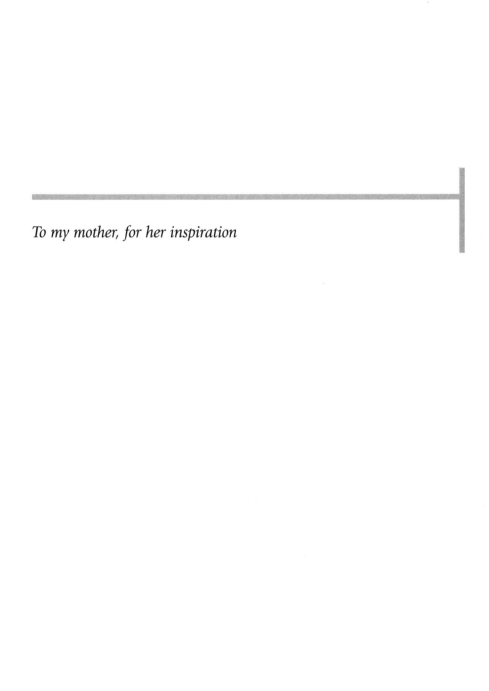

To my mother, for her inspiration

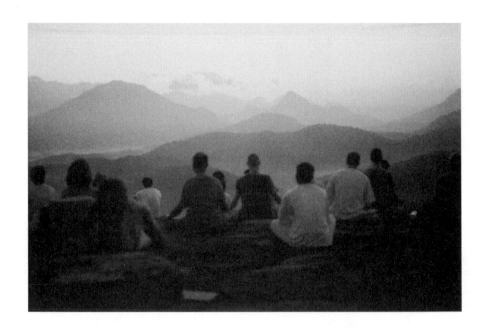

Contents

Foreword

The idea of anyone wanting to go to an ashram is both exotic and perplexing for most Americans. On the exotic side, we may have images of yogis with magical powers, out-of-body experiences, and blissful states of consciousness that we might hope to quickly gain for ourselves at the ashram. Others may look at an ashram as the home of some strange Eastern cult that should have no place in our modern scientific age, where we are likely to get brainwashed into leaving our family and job! Neither of these views is accurate. The spiritual experiences gained at an ashram usually result from long and patient work on oneself, and are more of peace and detachment than wild mystic adventures (though these can occur). Ashrams are places where we learn to decondition our minds and find our true selves, not where we are made into robots following any dogma or dictator.

Yet others may look at a yoga ashram like the yogic or Hindu equivalent of a religious retreat center, perhaps emphasizing some form of religious piety, study, or penance. This is not exactly accurate either. Ashrams are focused more on self-development, self-knowledge, and connection to the Divine within, rather than on a particular religious belief, scripture, or set of prayers and rituals on the outside. Yoga approaches God through nature and through healthy living, so the principles of health and general human happiness are likely to be taught as well.

Spiritual teachers from India have been a regular part of the American landscape for over a hundred years, since Swami Vivekananda first brought yoga and Vedanta to this country over a century ago. The interest in Hindu teachings is even older, with great American writers and thinkers such as Emerson and Thoreau drawing inspiration from the *Bhagavad Gita* and other Vedic teachings. Much of the recent interest in meditation in America has been due to the pioneering work of Indian teachers like Paramahansa Yogananda, Maharishi Mahesh Yogi, Muktananda, and others over the past several decades in this country.

Yoga has become an integral part of the American scene. While in our typical physical mindset we emphasize the exercise aspect of yoga, many yoga students are also looking at the religious and spiritual side of the tradition, including chanting, meditation, and the pursuit of a higher state of consciousness, which was more the original intent of yoga practice. This broader, spiritual approach to yoga is what ashrams have to offer.

Ashrams in India traditionally grew up around particular gurus and as places where their disciples, both mendicants and lay people, could come and receive teachings. Ashrams were usually located by temples or in beautiful natural settings, such as by mountains or the confluence of rivers. The ashram had its staff or residents largely responsible for its upkeep. This included resident students who studied closely with the teacher for an extended period. Small communities grew up around ashrams, including retirement homes and retreat houses.

This ashram model has come to the West as well. Most great yoga teachers from India have created such centers in this country. Here, where yogic practices are not supported by the general populace, ashrams have often turned into spiritual communities, having houses or facilities for residents, including married couples and families. However, some ashrams are still run mainly by monks or swamis and have no community directly attached to them.

Western ashrams are usually centered on various teaching programs, done on a daily, weekly, or monthly basis. These may include yoga teacher training, yoga philosophy, Ayurvedic medicine, Sanskrit, or chanting. Programs may include cultural events like music and dance, and outside speakers may be brought in to address a variety of topics, such as connecting yoga with science, medicine, and other important issues. This makes the Western ashram different from the Indian ashram, giving it its own flavor and an overall more interactive environment.

For his account, John Ittner uses an ashram with a long tradition both in the West and in India. It follows a lineage going back from Swami Vishnu-Devananda to Swami Sivananda of Rishikesh, one of modern India's greatest gurus and teachers of the past century.

The basic idea behind any ashram is that of *satsanga*, or the power of spiritual association. When we gather together for a common purpose we greatly augment the power of that purpose within each one of us. When we come together with spiritual intentions, the spiritual side of our nature is able to manifest in a much stronger way than if we were just attempting practices on our own. An ashram creates a kind of intensive or immersion training in yoga, in which yoga enters into one's daily life and personal interactions. One enters into a collective mindset aimed at inner growth that creates a favorable atmosphere for the soul to come forth. An important part of this is Karma Yoga, in which one helps with cooking and other community chores to be done along with a spirit of service.

Lighting the Lamp of Wisdom is a rare and insightful book about one person's honest experience inside a yoga ashram in the West. It is not an exposé by a scandal-mongering journalist or a dry academic account to fulfill a thesis requirement, but a lucid inside view by a person who has found deep value in the yoga tradition and in the ashram approach to spiritual life. The author's account is written in a colloquial style with much wit and humor, making it accessible to everyone and entertaining for anyone to read. He brings to life the characters and circumstances that come out in ashram settings, making readers feel that they are undergoing the ashram experience themselves.

Lighting the Lamp of Wisdom remedies any preconceptions one may have about ashram life, bringing it down to earth without losing its connection with the heavens. John Ittner shows ashram life as a meaningful spiritual and life experience that is open to everyone who aspires toward a greater contact with the Divine. The book is excellent reading for all those who want to broaden their appreciation of the human quest for higher truth. It is a good introduction to the deeper meaning and application of yoga.

> Dr. David Frawley (Pandit Vamadeva Shastri),
> author of *Yoga and Ayurveda, Yoga for
> Your Type,* and *Vedantic Meditation;*
> director, American Institute of Vedic Studies

Acknowledgments

Thanks must go to SkyLight Paths Publishing for its vision and skill. I am especially indebted to development editor Maura Shaw Tantillo, who felt that I was the right person to write this book. Maura helped me to stay focused, encouraged me to be myself, and kept my eye on the ball so that I could finish it on time. I also thank SkyLight Paths associate publisher Jon Sweeney for his support, and managing editor Emily Wichland for keeping the project rolling forward with a professional aplomb that is something like juggling.

Special thanks go to Srinivasan, director of the Sivananda Ashram Yoga Ranch, who supported this effort from inception to conclusion.

I conclude by thanking Swami Sivananda and Swami Vishnu-Devananda for all the Sivananda ashrams and centers around the world and for their enduring legacy of cultivating yoga.

Lighting the
Lamp of Wisdom

Introduction

With practice, within a few days, a little glimpse will
come, enough to give one encouragement and hope.

—SWAMI VIVEKANANDA

A week inside an ashram is like a peapod with seven peas in it. Each pea is round and perfect in itself, just like each day, but they still come from the same pod. There are seven chances to have the "little glimpse" promised by Swami Vivekananda. The daily ashram schedule has evolved over thousands of years. The schedule is designed to make it possible for you to be a yogi, even just for a day. That is enough to give you a real taste of the lifestyle and substance of that life. The symmetry of ending and beginning the day with meditation creates a frame and makes it easier to see the transformation that is happening. The seven peas turn into pearls all strung together by a thread of yoga. The ashram is the pod itself. It protects the peas so that they can focus on only one thing: growth.

The ashram is protection and nourishment. The first thing it protects you from is your lower self, not by telling you how terrible you are but by keeping your higher Self engaged all day in elevating situations. The ashram program has only one purpose: to open the way of a spiritual life. All you have to do is follow the schedule to see it work. The first obstacle the ashram overcomes is fear. This atmosphere of trust allows you to step outside your fortress and enjoy the world beyond the walls. Dropping the armor makes you feel light. Fear is one limiting factor that ashram life is designed to dissolve. Morning meditation paves the way for steady liberation throughout the day by enabling the mind to see itself at work. The two hours of *asana*s, or yoga postures, immediately following the meditation systematically bring the body into alliance with the breath. *Asana* class makes the body stronger and more flexible. You don't have to be a swami to notice the immediate benefits from *asana*s and *pranayama*, breath control exercises. When you are hungry, delicious simple food is served. Eating at the ashram is part ritual feast and part social event. Either way, the food is prepared according to Ayurvedic guidelines, and it plays a leading role in the change that is taking place. The ashram offers a chance to simplify your complex relationship with food. The discipline of waiting until you have completed meditation and *asana*s before eating ensures that your hunger is real. Food is put in its proper place. Discipline is rewarded, and you gain a "little glimpse."

Lest you become smug about how spiritual you have become with all the meditation and *asana*s, the ashram offers the perfect antidote: Karma Yoga. Karma Yoga is a no-brainer. At the minimum it offers you a chance to do something useful while digesting a healthy brunch. It's a good idea to move around after you eat anyway, so why not do a few chores around the ashram and meet your fellow guests and ashramites? You can get to know your neighbors and see what it takes to hold a utopian community together. Karma Yoga balances the day and offers you a chance to give something back. Already, you have received a lot. There is nothing selfish about meditating and doing *asana*s. In fact, they break down selfishness. But Karma Yoga is a chance to do something that directly matters. This is where the ideals of yoga meet the necessities of the real world. Swami Sivananda's far-flung influence is built on an edifice of selfless service by his disciple Swami Vishnu-Devananda. Now his disciples carry on the tradition. When you work with others at the ashram, you give service to a great enlightenment machine. When Swami Sivananda said "Work is worship," he opened the door for a new understanding. The feeling of being connected is always there when you work for others without thought of reward. Still, you know that you are creating some good karma—just enough to give you another "little glimpse."

When freedom comes at noon, we have already paid for it. This kind of freedom opens our eyes to the beauty that surrounds us. As human beings we are part of nature, but most of the time we never notice it. Now a whole morning has been spent knocking down walls—both interior and exterior, spiritual and physical, between us and nature. By now we are fairly defenseless and light as a dandelion seed, ready to be picked up by the wind and carried aloft. The sun is straight overhead. One-fourth of one day has passed. The baby pea is absorbing the maximum amount of nutrients from the pod. The ashram is nourishing our day to the fullest extent. Noon is a juicy-feeling time of day. Free time has just arrived. The discipline of the morning has begun to quiet the mind, but it has opened the senses and changed the nature of sensuality. The spiritual life is designed to refine our yearning for beauty by giving us finer pleasures. The process is inevitable. When I am walking up the hill to change for the sauna, and an Eastern bluebird flicks over my shoulder to join its flock in a budding oak, I chant, "Zippety-do-dah, zippety-ay." I just can't help it.

In the sauna the sweat beads up, and those beads turn into rivulets in the heat. The room is the color of freshly troweled cement and has a touch of the odor of curing concrete. This is reassuring—something like the new-car smell. It smells *sattwic*, clean. I see the drips hit the floor

and wonder how much toxin is really coming out. The muscles are suck-
ing up the heat. The more relaxed I am, the more heat I can take—and
the heat is way up there.

The second half of the day is like a mirror image of the first half.
You do it all again in nearly reverse order: the second half of the day is
more reflective; the first half was more expansive. Dinner is smaller than
brunch and not as festive. As the day winds down you begin to notice
that you are tired. The final meditation has a different flavor, tinged by
the events of the day and the dinner you just ate. You hear a lot of growl-
ing stomachs at evening *satsang,* a group session of meditation, chanting, and yoga. It's almost funny. When meditation ends, *Jaya Ganesha*
begins. The twenty-minute chant settles the stomachs and raises the
energy. In my experience, meditating after eating is harder, but chanting is easier. When the guard comes down the heart gets right in there
and takes advantage. The feeling behind the chants sinks straight in and
takes you with it. During the discussion of yoga philosophy, you might
think about bed—not because it is boring but because you are tired. The
absorption of Vedanta is an osmotic process at times. The day is not
completely finished until you lose consciousness of it in sleep. When
sleep takes over you never know what you will dream—but it doesn't
matter. What really matters is that sleep finishes making the pea in the
pod. If you are lucky, sleep will take you for a magic ride. Like a plant
you continue to grow in the night. Then the bell wakes you again, and
you start working on the next day. Each day is a little bit different from
the others but the days are more alike than different. When you have
seven of them all lined up like peas in a pod, you have a week inside an
ashram.

1

A Place for Grace

We've got to get ourselves back to the garden.

—JONI MITCHELL

The first day of the Yoga Teachers Training Course, we all lined up and took our turns at the microphone to answer a question. The question was "Why are you here?"

I wasn't sure I knew what to say, even though I had traveled ten time zones to get there. So I waited until almost the end to see what others would say. The obvious answer was that we were there to become certified yoga instructors. There were more than eighty of us, and we had come to the Sivananda Yoga Vedanta Dhanwantari Ashram in India's southern state of Kerala from all over the world. We had come from the United States, Canada, the United Kingdom, France, Germany, Switzerland, Belgium, Greece, Croatia, Chile, Malaysia, Cyprus, the Netherlands, Lebanon, South Africa, Singapore, Australia, New Zealand, Japan, Thailand, and India. We were like the United Nations of yoga.

As usual with yoga, there were a lot more women than men—about two out of three. Our ages ranged from the early twenties to nearly seventy, but the average age was about thirty, maybe a little younger. It's hard to tell with yogis because they often look younger than their real ages. We were racially, ethnically, and religiously diverse. On the surface we were all different, but our reasons for being here were not so different. No two people gave the same answer, but certain themes came up again and again. They boiled down to the fact that we all wanted to get in touch with our true nature. We wanted to get back to the Garden.

Not everyone expressed a desire to become a teacher. I'd guess that more than half ended up teaching. Wanting to teach sort of grew on you after you had tried it. Some already did teach; they wanted to dig deeper into the roots of yoga to become better teachers. Others wanted to perfect their postures; they couldn't get enough yoga outside of an ashram to suit them. Some said yoga had given them peace of mind, and they wanted more of that. Others wanted to go deeper into meditation. Some wanted to lose weight, look better, and feel younger (vanity is a big motivator). Some wanted to quit chasing their tails and get out of the rat race. Others had heard that the course was tough and were looking for a challenge. They had adventurous spirits and just wanted to give it a go. In most of us an inner voice whispered, "Follow your heart." When my turn came, I said I was there because I *needed* yoga. There were a few laughs, but the others knew what I was talking about. We all needed yoga. *Yoga* means "union with your higher Self." Who doesn't need that?

Cleaning Up Your Act

This was a lovely collection of people to begin with, and as the course went on it became even more so. The change was obvious on many levels. Yoga has the power to polish both the inner and the outer nature, and it shows. The mind becomes quieter, the eyes clearer. The skin and hair get glossier. The body becomes lighter and more flexible. The heart softens, and the intuition deepens. Looking back a year later on that wonderful month, I think that everyone got what she or he was looking for. Some got closer to their goals than others. That is not unusual—that's life. I am very happy to say that I got more than I had expected. As corny as it sounds, the Teachers Training Course was the gift that keeps on giving. Now I teach one class a week at the Sivananda Yoga Vedanta Center in New York City's Chelsea neighborhood. I am rewarded by seeing those Manhattanites walk into class tense and frowning and then see them leave relaxed and smiling. It never fails. There is a saying that for every step you take toward God, God takes fifty steps toward you. This is true whether you believe in God or not. To go to an ashram is to take that step. Then watch out!

Some of the reasons why people came were spoken that day, and some were left unsaid. You tend to put the best face on things when you are talking to scores of people you hardly know. The sharing of ashram life opens people's hearts. If you listen, you can learn a lot about them in a short time, especially if you are open yourself. There may be a broken heart from a love affair, or a marriage that has fallen apart. Sometimes there has been a death of someone near and dear. A drug or alcohol problem may make someone want to avoid certain people and places. Another person might have lost a job. Getting fired can be a shattering experience, but depending on the person's responsibilities, it can create an opening to break away from a numbing routine.

Thanks to the phenomenal growth of yoga, ashrams are very trendy these days—and you will find a lot of trendy people, too. That is a good thing. It's about time. Yoga may be thousands of years old, but suddenly it is an overnight success. The media portrays ashrams as expensive and exclusive enclaves where movie stars and rock musicians look absolutely fabulous in leotards, where the rich and famous drop in, work out, eat healthy food, go to bed early, say hello to God, and dry out if they need to get away from temptation. Ashrams often are seen as sanctuaries for seekers of sacred novelties or as halfway houses for rebellious youths trying to run away from the religion of their birth.

Roar Like Your Real Self

Going to an ashram is like going to work, but you are working on yourself. That is the important difference, other than the fact that you are not paid. You will pay off some karmic debts, but that is another matter. The job, instead of being outside of you, *is* you. Whatever you put in, you will get back; so there is no point in slacking off. You are the one who will enjoy the fruits of your labor. Yoga is a wonderfully efficient system, but it takes some time to get used to it. Maybe all this focus on the self sounds selfish to you. What about others? Don't they matter? Of course they do.

Now is a good time to make an important distinction. You come to an ashram to work toward finding your eternal spiritual Self. The ashram is designed so that you can spend the whole day looking for something that you already have. That sounds strange, but it goes to the heart of ashram life, just as this vision of the Self with a capital S goes to the heart of yoga. This Self is sacred because it is the soul. In fact, this Self, or *Atman,* is one with God—our true nature. Yogis call this Self-realization *Sat-chid-ananda*: Existence, Knowledge, and Bliss Absolute.

A story told by yogis helps illustrate this Self-realization. A shepherd tending his flock heard a prowling lion and shot at it. The lion was a female and very pregnant. Startled by the shot, she was running away when the baby popped out. The sheep heard the cries of the baby and took it to live with them. They nursed it and taught it to eat grass and to bleat "baa, baa, baa." The lion cub started learning the ways of sheep.

One day when the sheep were grazing, a big lion came. He was incensed to see a noble lion cub eating grass and bleating like a sheep. All the sheep were scared to death and ran away—all except for the young lion. The big lion was annoyed with the sheep-lion. He asked him why he was eating grass like sheep. Sheep-lion bleated, "What are you talking about? I am a sheep." The lion said, "Come with me." He took the baby lion to the edge of a still lake and told him to look at the reflection in the water. "What do you see?" he asked. "Do you see a sheep?" The baby lion looked in the water and saw his face for the first time. Suddenly a feeling of tremendous well-being came over him. The lion saw it and said, "Now let's hear you roar." The young lion opened his mouth, and a roar came out. He liked it so well that he kept on roaring. The moral is this: we are all lions who have forgotten our true divine nature.

The lion who showed the sheep-lion his reflection in the water acted as a guru does. *Guru* means "remover of darkness." What could be darker than going around certain that you are a sheep when you are really a lion? That story was a favorite of one of India's great gurus, Himalayan yoga master Swami Sivananda, and of his disciple Swami Vishnu-Devananda. In 1957, with ten rupees in his pocket, as the story goes, Swami Vishnu left India for the West. His master sent him with these words: "People are waiting!" Swami Vishnu-Devananda traveled across the Pacific. Landing in San Francisco, he crossed the continent, lecturing and teaching yoga wherever he stopped. He was a young lion himself: thirty years old, fearless, tireless, brilliant, and enthusiastic. He knew the secrets of Hatha Yoga, the kind of physical self-mastery that Westerners were hungry to know, and he knew how to share his knowledge so that people could understand him.

Swami Vishnu-Devananda's training under Swami Sivananda had given him the tools he needed to introduce yoga on a large scale. He had been Swami Sivananda's personal secretary. He had managed the ashram's kitchen, overseen building projects, and worked in publishing. He was best known as Hatha Yoga professor of the Yoga Vedanta Forest Academy. The pliability of his body and his ability to perform yoga postures was as legendary as his energy. He was courageous and irrepressible in his enthusiasm. In 1959, he opened his first permanent yoga center in Montreal, Canada. Although it thrived, he noticed that class attendance fell off in the summer months. When he asked why, he was told that in the summer the citizens of Montreal went north to the Laurentian Mountains for summer vacations. He saw people coming back from their normal getaways more exhausted than when they left. They ate too much, drank and smoked, stayed up late, and woke up with hangovers. They literally wore themselves out trying to have fun. When it was all over, they worried about how much money they had spent. In a typical flash of inspiration, Swami Vishnu-Devananda had a vision: "Why not create a yoga vacation?"

In the summer of 1963, he opened the first yoga camp in the Laurentian Mountains north of Montreal. This collection of small buildings and tents became the first permanent yoga retreat in the Western Hemisphere. He was amazed how hungry people in the West were for yoga. They would sleep on the floor or in tents and take cold showers, all in the hope of spiritual growth and physical well-being from yoga. His yoga vacation idea became very popular, and by 1975 he had established three more ashrams: on Paradise Island in the Bahamas; in Grass Valley, California; and at the Yoga Ranch in New York's Catskill Mountains.

Long and Winding Road to Yoga

They say there is no such thing as a coincidence, that what happens was meant to happen. If that is true, and I believe it is, I have a lot of thanks to give Swami Vishnu-Devananda for how I got started in yoga. A great yogi generates a force field that carries far even after he has passed from this earth.

When I was a senior in high school, I was captain of the wrestling team. One of my teammates lived next door to me, and after school I used to hang out at his house. His mother took ten different kinds of vitamins and frequented health food stores. One day she gave me a book she thought I would like: *Yoga, Youth, and Reincarnation.* I loved rough contact sports, but I was also secretly fascinated by religion and mysticism, and the book turned me on. I followed the instructions in the book and taught myself to stand on my head. I also took a fancy to gazing into candle flames. The author, Jess Stearn, was a *New York Daily News* feature writer. He had found a guru, and that woman's guru was Swami Vishnu-Devananda. Stearn's book was based on a stay at her ashram. Her teaching was largely what she had learned from Swamiji. (*Swamiji* is a term of endearment and respect that a yogi gives to a *sannyasin,* one who has taken the vows to be celibate.) I didn't realize the connection until recently, when I picked up the book again to remind myself of what I had liked so much about it. When I read the reference to Swami Vishnu, it made sense. Then (to really speed up my story), Vietnam came along, and I went into the navy to stay out of the army. College and marriage followed, and I forgot about yoga—or at least I thought I had forgotten. Yoga has a way of staying alive inside of you without your knowing it.

Yoga returned to my life about ten years later in the early 1980s. I was living on the Upper West Side of Manhattan, divorced with no children, and working at the *New York Post* as a copy editor. One day I spotted a sign in a second-floor window on West 72nd Street advertising yoga classes. I remembered how much I had liked standing on my head and gazing at candles, so I called the number and started taking real classes for the first time. The style of yoga taught there was Iyengar, named after B. K. S. Iyengar, author of the classic Hatha Yoga book *Light on Yoga,* which has served as an important guidebook for countless practitioners. I was fortunate to have as teachers two dedicated and inspired women who functioned like the good cop and the bad cop. One was gentle and the other was forceful. They taught on different days, but together they made a great team, like yin and yang. Their spiritual names were Rudrani and Rama. At first I wondered what their real names were. A new name seemed to me like a big commitment. Between the two of them I made some progress. The Iyengar method of teaching puts great emphasis on getting the postures absolutely correct, and I received a strong foundation there. Props such as wooden blocks and straps were used to hold the student in the right position. Rama and Rudrani taught me how to feel the balance, scan the body for tension, and visualize myself holding the *asana*s, as the yoga postures are called. They understood the fine line between making a strong effort to get into more advanced postures and not injuring yourself by overdoing it. A basic precept in yoga, called *ahimsa* in Sanskrit, means "noninjury." It means not to kill or hurt any living being. That is one of the reasons why yogis do not eat meat. The principle also applies to our own *asana* practice: with awareness we can keep from hurting ourselves. "Be brave but careful" is a good rule. Listen to your body.

I was enjoying the *asana*s and occasionally found myself meditating, but I was unschooled in the devotional side of yoga, called Bhakti Yoga. One afternoon at the end of class, Rudrani, the nice cop, told me that she was going upstate to the SYDA (Siddha Yoga Dham of America) Foundation ashram in the Catskills for what was called an "Intensive" weekend. She thought I would like it, too, but if I wanted to go I should decide quickly, as they tended to completely fill up. Rudrani was a follower of Guru Mayi, a young Indian swami, who was then in her twenties. She had been chosen to lead the organization founded by her guru, Swami Muktananda, after he had passed on. I was intrigued at the thought of spending a weekend at an ashram and seeing a real guru. "Guru Mayi" means "guru mother." I thought "Intensive" had a nice ring to it. It sounded, well, intense. Having no real idea about what I was in for, I made a reservation that day. That weekend was twenty years ago, and I still remember it well. We were driven upstate in a full charter bus. Every seat was taken. The SYDA compound on the outskirts of South Fallsburg, New York, was so large that there was a smaller shuttle bus to take us from the check-in building to the temple and dormitories. The SYDA compound seemed almost as big as the town. This was the first ashram I had ever seen, and I was impressed.

The SYDA Foundation was superbly organized. At check-in we all had our pictures taken and were issued photo identification cards that looked like driver's licenses, only prettier. We were instructed to wear them at all times. At first I wasn't sure that I liked this, but the tags made it easy to remember names. I knew no one so this was helpful. I was assigned a room with three other guys. There were two bunk beds. It felt like summer camp, but it was bigger and nicer. To my surprise, yoga *asanas* were not on the schedule for those of us participating in the "Intensive." Hatha Yoga classes were offered on an optional basis, but there was not a lot of time for them. Instead, we attended scheduled chanting sessions, called *kirtan*, and lectures in a huge auditorium. The cafeteria, staffed by cheerful volunteers, was larger than I had expected. The food was plentiful and healthful, though a bit bland to my taste. Those who did not care for the cafeteria food could use a separate eatery where there was more choice, but at an extra charge.

We were assigned numbered areas on the floor of the auditorium, which was marked off into sections of about one square yard for each person. My square yard was mine for the whole weekend. At the back of the auditorium were normal theater seats for older people and anyone else who did not want to sit for hours on the floor. The auditorium was grand, with large colored chandeliers. After the lecture the lights would be dimmed, and we would begin to chant "Om" together. The vibration that came from that auditorium with thousands of devotees was overwhelming. It could make me cry. This "Intensive" lived up to its name. Large feelings welled up in my chest during the chanting. My voice was like a drop of water in an ocean of emotion. I merged into the moment, into a zone.

The weekend climaxed on Sunday with a ceremony in which we all

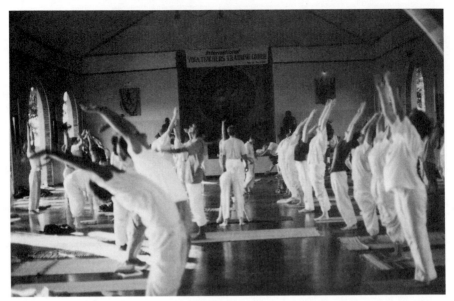

Hatha Yoga classes at the ashram in Kerala, India, were held in the open-air hall twice a day. The floor was smoothly polished black marble tile that was always clean and cool to the touch.

lined up and, one after the other, bowed before Guru Mayi, who was sitting on a "throne." She wore her orange robes like a queen. I couldn't help wondering what it would be like to kiss her. This says more about my state of mind twenty years ago than about her. She was only in her twenties but was already being worshiped like a saint. When she spoke, her voice sounded wise but playful. Hundreds of us waited to receive *shaktipat* from her. This blessing, which can be given by a guru, is the awakening of the *kundalini shakti:* the name of the coiled serpent power that resides in the lower spinal area and is dormant in most of us. When this power rises up a channel in the spinal cord called the *shushumna nadi* and reaches an area at the top of the skull called the *sahasrara chakra,* we experience *samadhi,* or enlightenment. I did not know what I was doing, but I hoped that she did.

As we prostrated she brushed our backs with a bundle of peacock feathers to awaken this power. I had never bowed before a person before, and doing it made me uncomfortable. Worshiping a person, even a guru, is not the way I was brought up. I was curious, though, and hopeful that she had real power to enlighten me. I did not think that I had any particular right to such a gift, but I would not turn down such an opportunity. So I smiled and bowed, hoping she would give me whatever she could give. When the peacock feathers touched my back, I felt a pleasant sensation. The change might have been too subtle for my understanding. I felt spiritually high from chanting and thought that Guru Mayi had a shiny aura—a deeply compassionate beauty that was inspiring. No one could deny that many of those she touched were deeply moved.

Back in Manhattan, my yoga practice waned as I slowly worked my way up the totem pole at the *New York Post*. From my lowly beginning as a copy boy I became the news editor. Now I was responsible for getting the paper out every night by deadline and helping decide what was news and what wasn't. I also supervised the layout and composition of the news pages in the front of the paper and wrote as many front-page headlines as I could. My most famous headline was "WACKO JACKO BACKO." No *Post* headline will ever top the classic "HEADLESS BODY IN TOPLESS BAR," but we tried. Every evening at six we had a meeting of the most senior editors, when we would duke it out to see who could come up with the best headline—the one that would scream loudly enough to get someone to cross the street and buy the paper.

I was proud of my job, but bit by bit my heart was getting harder. The gallows humor at a newspaper can be as hilarious as the subject matter is tragic. Humor is a very powerful defense mechanism and a necessity for newspaper editors. There was a hollow feeling inside me that I was trying to fill with bad habits and that eventually became obvious to those closest to me. Most nights I worked until eleven o'clock or midnight. They say New York is the city that never sleeps, and that is true. What that really means is that the bars don't close until 4 A.M.

Swami Vishnu re-entered my life when a truly fine friend did what only a good friend can do. He told me he thought it would be a good idea for me to spend a weekend at an ashram. He didn't say, "I think you need to get yourself straightened out." He didn't have to say that because I knew it as well as anybody, but he did something about it. He went online and found the Sivananda Yoga Ranch Ashram and made reservations for two, and he even came with me. We rode up in the ashram's van from the city, and I liked the ashram so well that I came back the next three weekends in a row. I even wrote a story about it that ran in the *Post*, where I called it "yoga boot camp." The first sentence of the piece read thus: "The night before I went to the ashram I drank ten beers at the Corner Bistro, ordered a hamburger at 3 A.M., and bummed a Camel Light from the bartender." I was told that after the story ran, the ashram got a lot of calls from people asking, "Is this the yoga boot camp?"

Meanwhile, Back at the Ranch

Every Friday at 6 P.M., a white passenger van leaves the Sivananda Yoga Vedanta Center on West 24th Street in Manhattan and heads upstate to the ashram in the Catskills. The trip from the city to the Yoga Ranch is always difficult at the beginning. The journey of about a hundred miles lasts approximately three hours because it takes so long to get out of the city on Fridays, when everybody else is also trying to get out of town. Without fail, there is bumper-to-bumper traffic for most of the first hour. I have now made this trip many times and have come to see it as a meditation, a chance to slow down and leave my cares behind. Three hours is long enough to calm the restless mind. The Chinese say that a journey of a thousand miles begins with a single step.

When I sit down to meditate, my mind is overflowing with thoughts competing for my attention. They are like honking horns—impossible to ignore. Trying to clear my mind of thoughts is like getting through rush-hour traffic. In meditation I learned to let the thoughts come and drift away like clouds in a clear blue sky. Even honking horns come and go. After a while I begin to observe my thoughts with a certain detachment instead of obsessing on them. The first time I took the van to the ashram, I felt very frustrated by the traffic. Even now, when I meditate I'm thinking about how my back is stiff, my legs hurt, and my feet are going to sleep. My mind races along at its usual frenetic pace, but if I keep my attention on the breath I forget about it. When I least expect it, I notice that I have slipped into a deeper awareness. In traffic terms, I have left the city behind. I am now on the George Washington Bridge soaring high over the majestic Hudson River. Like my mind, the city is still there. I can see it by looking over my shoulder. It's not in my face. I feel my attention drawn to my fellow passengers. The positive energy and the forced proximity in the crowded van make conversation easy. The ashram beckons in the distance. I can feel it. Excitement is in the air, and it shows in the faces around me. There is an awareness that we are about to share an adventure. Social and psychological barriers begin to ease because there is a shared purpose of an elevating sort. We are going on a spiritual trip. We have made a date with our higher Self.

Finally we arrive at the ashram, and what we see is a turn-of-the-century white clapboard farmhouse with a modern temple grafted onto one side. There is nothing very grand about it, but it sits on top of a high hill with miles and miles of views, and it oozes serenity. Up the hill are two red three-story dormitory buildings the size and shape of dairy barns. They were built in the 1940s, when this was Bel Air Hotel, known for its fresh air. In one incarnation it was a dude ranch. Like many other spiritual establishments in the southern Catskills, the Sivananda Yoga Ranch uses buildings that date to the Borscht Belt era, when a largely Jewish clientele would escape New York City for some fresh air, family fun, horseback riding, a little golf, some tennis and swimming, good food, and nightclub entertainers. In its heyday from the 1940s to the 1960s, the Borscht Belt was a popular destination. But times change, and as the clientele became more affluent and flights became cheaper, they took vacations in Florida or Europe. The Borscht Belt—spawning ground of some of comedy's big names such as George Carlin, Alan King, and Danny Kaye—became itself a joke. One by one the resorts closed down. Many of them are still empty, but in the 1970s, religious groups started buying them for retreats. The prices were right, and the location was still good for these fixer-uppers. Just add work—a lot of it—and you had an instant ashram, or meditation center. They don't look particularly religious on the outside, but they work. Some clever magazine writer rechristened this area the Buddha Belt, and the name stuck.

The farmhouse is rustic and the temple is modern. Somehow they harmonize. Temple and farmhouse are like two happily married people that no one would have expected to wed because they look too different from each other. You would not expect them to get along, but they do. He's a farm boy and she's an Indian princess. It's the attraction of opposites. Like America and yoga, they love each other.

When I arrive by van, supper is waiting, but first I must check in. This procedure at the ashram is not much different from checking into a hotel. It requires either a credit card or cash. The price at this time— $55 a night for a shared room on the weekend—includes two meals a day and two Hatha Yoga classes. The rooms are simple and homey. Most have two narrow beds, a chest of drawers, a bedside table, and a lamp. Each room has a copy of Swami Vishnu's *Meditation and Mantras* and *The Sivananda Ashram Guest Handbook* on the table. All the Sivananda ashrams run on the same daily schedule, whether in India; upstate New York; Grass Valley, California; Paradise Island in the Bahamas; Neuville aux Bois outside of Paris; or the Tyrolean Alps of Austria. The only thing that changes is the time zone and the view.

2

Complete Immersion

God has arranged for many ways of worship to suit the various temperaments of God's worshipers in their different stages of growth.

—SRI RAMAKRISHNA

The wake-up bell rings at 5:30 A.M., but it is as dark outside as the middle of the night. I know this because I have opened one eye. I wish I could say that I always bounce out of bed, but sometimes I do. Getting adjusted to the ashram schedule takes some time. How I wake up depends on how well I sleep. Everyone is different, but I find that it takes about three days to get used to waking up in the dark. Until then the morning bell comes as a shock. After a while at the ashram I need less sleep to be fully rested. Swami Sivananda said that yogis should sleep about six hours. He considered too much sleep to be *tamasic,* lazy. One reason the ashram day starts so early is that the early morning hours are considered especially good for meditation. As night shifts into day there is a time of balance, a sacred pause called *Brahmamuhurta,* said by yogis to be *sattwic,* a time of balance and peace when meditation comes more easily. As for waking up, at first I find it painful, but by the end of a week it is joyful. The *Bhagavad Gita* says, "That which is like poison at first, but in the end like nectar—that happiness is declared to be *sattwic,* born of the purity of one's own mind due to Self-realization."

With the help of vigorous bell ringing, the ashram runs on time. For every event of the day, the bell ringing sets off a different reaction. At 5:30 A.M. it is disbelief. At 7:50 A.M. it is anticipation of *asana* class. At 9:50 A.M., hungry for breakfast, we salivate like Pavlov's dogs.

Wake-up duty is a form of Karma Yoga. A member of the ashram staff has to get up first and get everyone else up. In case I miss the bell, a more surgical strike comes soon after in the form of a gong being pounded briskly in the hall outside the door. The gong sounds weirdly theatrical for that time of day, as if we are getting up to perform on stage. Eventually, even the gong goes away. If I close my eyes again, the next twenty minutes pass in what seems like twenty seconds. The ten-minute warning bell gets me out of the sack, knowing that I have only ten minutes before meditation begins in the temple. As much as I enjoy sleeping, I hate being late for *satsang* and missing the meditation. I rush through the morning self-cleansing ritual. I wash my feet, hands, and face. I brush my teeth and put on clean clothes. These are called temple rules. When I follow them I am more *sattwic.* The word, which means pure, or clear, is derived from the Sanskrit *sattwa* and describes a state wherein nature is in balance and the mind sees unity and truth. Meditation experience confirms that "cleanliness is next to godliness." They just seem to go together.

Outside the temple doors, a sign is posted requesting silence for the ten minutes preceding the meditation. The sign is posted because ashram guests tend to gather there until the last minute, and some people are already meditating in the temple. The temple is entered from a hall between the farmhouse and the temple. This hall is wide enough for chairs and sofas and serves as the ashram's axis—its major highway, artery, and hangout. It runs from the front door to a mud room to a sitting room with a wood stove, and ends at the tearoom. It is also the favorite of the ashram cats, Bikshu and Nandi, whose beds flank the stove. In the winter, a crowd forms around the stove, and the cats soak up the warmth and attention. People with sleepy faces burn their tongues with hot tea to wake up outside the temple doors.

Company of the Wise

The ashram day begins with meditation, chanting, and a talk about yoga. This gathering is called *satsang,* which means "company of the wise." It is basically a religious service. There are two *satsangs* every day: one from 6:00 to 7:30 in the morning and the other from 8:00 until 9:30 in the evening. *Satsangs* are major ashram events, and attendance is considered mandatory. At Sivananda ashrams, *satsang* is first on the schedule in the morning and the last event at night before bedtime. The morning and evening *satsangs* are the heart of the ashram experience. These rituals create a sacred space between them and set the tone for everything that follows. Ashram life can be understood as a series of rituals designed to lift the awareness to a higher level and keep it there.

Satsang is mandatory at Sivananda ashrams to ensure that visitors will be able to experience the transforming power of yoga. They need to participate in the rituals to get the full effect. When people take a holiday, they often sleep late, but anyone who sleeps until ten o'clock at the ashram misses half the day. The way to have the best possible ashram experience is to join in and keep an open mind. There is ancient knowledge behind these practices, and those who open up can absorb some of it. This is especially true of *satsangs,* which are easily the most foreign events in the day for Westerners. At *satsang* we practice three kinds of yoga. First, we meditate; this is a form of Raja Yoga in which we work on concentrating the mind. Second, we chant; this is Bhakti Yoga, the path of love and devotion to God. The *satsang* ends with a talk about Vedanta, the philosophy of yoga. This path is called Jnana Yoga, which uses the power of the mind to sort out the difference between the eternal and that which changes. By practicing all three, one prepares the way for progress in all aspects of yoga. These three yogas support one another, deepening the experience. Bhakti Yoga engages the heart and keeps the Jnana Yoga from getting stuck in the head. Raja Yoga meditation without devotion is less powerful than it is with devotion. When people worship together there is a sharing, and everyone gets more out of it. Everyone's presence at *satsang* makes a difference.

I go straight into the temple with three minutes to spare. On this Saturday morning the temple is almost full. There are about twenty guests, plus about ten staff members. This is a decent showing for midwinter. On the summer weekends there can be sixty or more guests, and on holidays there may be a hundred or more. Entering the temple is like entering another world, a sacred space where only one thing really matters—discovering the God that is inside me. Everything about *satsang* is for the purpose of enhancing this experience of inner silence. I kneel to the altar and sit on a cushion with my legs crossed. The idols on the altar seem to glow in the dim light. Fresh flowers flank them. An oil lamp gives a steady yellowish light in the bluish predawn. The incense wafts through the still air. As I shut my eyes the temple doors open behind me, and the latecomers enter. I can hear them trying not to make any noise. The rustling, the coughing, and the clearing of throats take a couple of minutes to settle down.

Sometimes meditation is easy. Other times the mind has a mind of its own. The mind is so hard to control that Swami Vishnu sometimes compared it to a drunken monkey that has been stung by a scorpion. It cannot be kept from wandering, and it has to be watched. The only solution is to gently keep bringing it back. As sound dies away I feel a change in the atmosphere, and calm prevails. In the peaceful morning we are touched by the silence. Having touched the silence, we want to dive deeper.

Sometimes, when my mind is restless, I open my eyes and gaze at the altar for a couple of minutes. Then I close my eyes again and try to meditate. When I close my eyes, the idols on the altar remain for a moment as afterimages. They help to hold the mind steady. Like people, the idols wear different garments from day to day. There is a devotional ritual called *puja* in which the idols are lovingly dressed by a priest or members of the ashram staff. This Bhakti Yoga practice is one of the subtle touches the staff adds to the ashram atmosphere. Just as a child plays the role of an adoring mother with her dolls, the devotee ceremonially acts out here the love of God. It is said by Patanjali in his *Yoga-Sutras* that devotion is the easiest way to cultivate concentration and meditation.

The meditation ends when Srinivasan, the director of the Yoga Ranch, breaks the silence with "Om." We repeat the sacred syllable three times. When I open my eyes the early morning darkness has turned into light. Some darkness in me is also dispelled, and I too am lighter. Meditation seems to end at about the time when I have forgotten that I've been meditating. At the end of the meditation I was no longer aware of my body. The change is subtle and softening, but my foot has fallen asleep and feels as if it belongs to someone else. I massage it to get the blood moving again. When the lights are turned on at 6:30, my mind is refreshed and deeply relaxed. It is time to chant.

Singing the Names of the Lord

Srinivasan slides his gently battered harmonium to a position in front of his lap and plays the opening chord to the familiar *Jaya Ganesha*. At Sivananda ashrams every *kirtan* begins like this. The chanting of *Jaya Ganesha* brings a welcome change from sitting in silence. The atmosphere in the temple evolves from solemn to joyous when the chanting begins. The *prana* starts pumping, and the spirit moves to the sound of the mantras. Various drums, tambourines, bells, and other percussion instruments are passed out to accompany the chanting. Some people clap their hands. It is said that in ancient times the *rishis*, or saints, developed *kirtan* as one way to control the mind and bring the mind's focus to the Divine. *Kirtan* is singing God's name with devotion, or *bhava*. It is said that chanting the name of the Lord soothes the nerves, turns the emotions in a positive direction, and purifies the heart. Even so, many people find it strange at first.

This chant begins with a mantra hailing the elephant-headed god, Ganesha, and asking for his protection. Ganesha is worshiped as a remover of obstacles. Nothing gets in his way. Because there are so many obstacles in our way to success in both the spiritual and the physical worlds, he is very popular. We need to remove the obstacles just to get started. There is something jolly about his image as well. He is non-threatening and lovable, like Babar the Elephant. It is said that his image embodies the primordial word "Om." Just as many chants begin with "Om," many chants also begin by giving homage to Ganesha.

The purpose of chanting is to create a pure vibration that can open the heart. The chanting works best when the chanter pronounces the Sanskrit words correctly with devotion and awareness of the meaning. The sound of the mantra is said to be the embodiment of God. In the first chapter of the Gospel of John in the New Testament, the first line says, "In the beginning was the Word, and the Word was God." That sounds like the definition of a mantra. With this in mind, let us go through the translation of *Jaya Ganesha* step by step. By understanding this seminal chant, we can learn something about what is considered important in this form of worship. For the sake of brevity, I will not include the Sanskrit words that are actually chanted but rather focus on what they mean.

The chant begins by saying "victory to Ganesha." It asks him to save and protect us. He is not only the remover of obstacles but also the god of new beginnings. At the beginning of a new day or a new venture, it is considered auspicious to ask his help. The verses that follow invoke Subramanya, the leader of the army of the gods, asking him to help drive off all demons and negative influences. Next, Saraswati, patroness of arts and learning, is saluted. Saraswati bestows intuition, intelligence, self-control, and success in deep subjects. The guru, who is seen as God, is hailed next for giving the teachings that lead to bliss and knowledge. The *Maha Mantra*, or Great Mantra, is then sung in praise of Ram and Krishna. This is among the most powerful of all the mantras and is best known as *Hare Krishna*. It bestows purity to the heart and the mind. Next, the guru Swami Sivananda and his disciple Swami Vishnu-Devananda have their turn. This is followed by the mantra to Siva, the destroyer of evil and the first and greatest of all the gurus. Then Vishnu, the preserver of the universe, is celebrated with his mantra. The repetition of this very powerful mantra is said to bring infinite peace, mercy, and goodness. This mantra is chanted daily at the ashram to create a vibration that helps bring peace to the world. Next to be hailed is Vasudeva, another name for Krishna. It is Krishna who bestowed the most valuable of all Vedantic texts, the *Bhagavad Gita*, to humankind. Then Swami Sivananda and Swami Vishnu-Devananda are once more invoked, followed by praises to Ram, who is God in the form of the ideal man, and to Hanuman, the monkey god who personifies devotion. The next two mantras invoke Dattatreya and Sankaracharya, two great gurus of *advaita* (nondualistic) Vedanta. As we approach the end, Krishna is hailed once more, and the chant finally ends with a mantra invoking Siva.

After a week in an ashram, parts of this chant become embedded in the unconscious mind. The tune is as simple as a child's song, and there are not very many words. Some mantras are short and sweet, capable of being repeated with one breath, and others are long. At first, *Jaya Ganesha* is incomprehensible—just a series of sounds—but after a while the words become more familiar. If you stay at the ashram for a week and attend all the *satsangs*, you will have chanted *Jaya Ganesha* fourteen times. At about twenty minutes apiece, that adds up to about four hours on this chant alone. There is an English translation in the book, but at first it is hard to follow it while trying to pronounce all the unfamiliar Sanskrit words. The best way to learn the proper pronunciation is to read the words as you chant them and read the translation at another time. Eventually you will know them. That is where the repetition comes in: after a while you quit worrying about it and just do it. Then it starts to feel good. All this repetition reminds me of the movie *Groundhog Day*, in which Bill Murray keeps waking up over and over again to Sonny and Cher singing "I Got You, Babe." I find this movie to be a fair analogy for the ritual of ashram life. You do the same things over and over again. You follow the same rituals in the same order. The only thing that changes is you.

Giving Chants a Chance

There is a wide range of feelings among first-time visitors on the subject of chanting. Some dive right in and love it immediately. Other people say they find the Sanskrit confusing. They are bothered by not knowing what the chants mean. They worry about praising gods they have never heard of. This problem seems to be larger for some than for others. Some people may also be bothered that attendance at *satsang* is required. They came for the *asanas* and got religion. There are places to go for those who would prefer to practice *asanas* and eat healthy food in lovely surroundings and not mix religion into it, but they are spas and not ashrams. Most people at the ashram are open-minded on the subject. They do not object to the devotional aspect of yoga. One big reason people come to an ashram for the first time is to become aligned with a higher power, to make their lives more spiritual. They are prepared for something different from the familiar. They want a break from the limitations of everyday life. Those who give themselves permission to chant with an open heart, without fear that they are slighting the religious tradition into which they were born, often find themselves enjoying it. That enjoyment turns out to be the first step to deeper knowledge of what it means to praise the Lord, whether in the form of Jesus, Jehovah, Buddha, or any other god. For me, sometimes chanting is like the magic moment when disbelief has been suspended and the characters in a movie come to life, only more powerfully. This is purely personal, but I have felt closer to the divine power when chanting than when meditating.

I am one of those people who tried to follow the words and join in even without knowing what they meant. I remember stumbling through the verses and thinking that I did not have a clue. Having been brought up as a Christian, I wondered if Jesus would hear these prayers and be offended—jealous maybe. There was a picture of Jesus on the wall behind the altar in the ashram's temple, but there is no Ganesha on the altar of any church I have ever attended. I would still put myself in the category of those who feel that they do not understand exactly what it all means. Having heard and chanted *Jaya Ganesha* many times, I am still changing the way I feel about it. Since it works for me, I give chanting of mantras the benefit of the doubt. It was the hardest yoga practice to feel comfortable about at first, but it did not contradict my understanding of the teachings of Christ. Through experience I had gained faith in all the yogic practices I had tried, so it was easy for me to give chanting a chance. I had already experienced the health benefits of *asana* practice and the yogic diet. Having seen for myself that ashram life was healthy and positive, I saw nothing to fear in chanting. Now, when I worship in a church, I have an enriched appreciation of singing hymns, and I enjoy singing them even more. From my days of singing in the church choir, I have always felt that music was the most direct way to feel the presence of God.

Now I look forward to *kirtan*. I love the way it wakes me up and gets the blood going after meditation. It is a chance to praise God directly, which is something of a relief after a long silent meditation of looking within. During the morning chants I become more and more awake. Swami Sivananda, who said there were many paths to God, called *kirtan* the easiest, surest, and quickest way to God-realization in the difficult times in which we live. Swami Vishnu liked to joke that it was also the cheapest.

According to Vedanta, this period in which we now live is called the *Kali Yuga,* or Iron Age. A Hindu scripture written 5,000 years ago, the *Srimad Bhagavatam,* described this era in a way that is strikingly accurate. Among other things, it says, "In the Kali Age wealth alone will be the criteria of social status, morality and merit. . . . Might will be the only factor determining righteousness and fairness. . . . Trickery alone will be the motive force in business dealings. . . . Hypocrisy will replace goodness. . . . Femininity and masculinity will be judged solely on the ability to perform well sexually," and so on. This does sound like our time, does it not? If *kirtan* can help us through all that, I feel that there is nothing wrong with giving it a chance.

Jaya Ganesha is always the first chant, but it is never the last. After it is finished, two or three more mantras will be chanted, usually led by staff members, who will choose their favorites. I have noticed that people who have taken spiritual names such as Krishna or Shakti will often choose a chant to invoke that deity. These secondary chants add variety to the *satsang.* Some of them are old favorites that regular ashram visitors have come to know, and others are more obscure, known by only a few.

Images and Idols on the Altar

Chanting is followed by a talk on the practice and philosophy of yoga. In a recent talk, Srinivasan addressed the meaning of the idols on the altar. Getting accustomed to the altar takes some time. There are so many elements that visitors can be confused. After three years of coming to the ashram I was still not sure about the meaning of some of the statues and pictures. So I was very glad when Sri (his nickname) took up the subject. I had been concerned at first that I was worshiping idols, and the first commandment of the Hebrew scripture clearly states, "Thou shalt not put any other gods before me." I did not know how to feel about worshiping at an altar that had lots of gods on it. There was a picture of Jesus, but it seemed strange to see him in the same context as Hanuman, the monkey god, Krishna playing his flute, or Swami Sivananda.

Srinivasan is a tall man, and he looks even taller when he is sitting down because he sits up so straight. In his late forties, he looks younger, like a college professor with angular, even features and kind eyes. Sri has

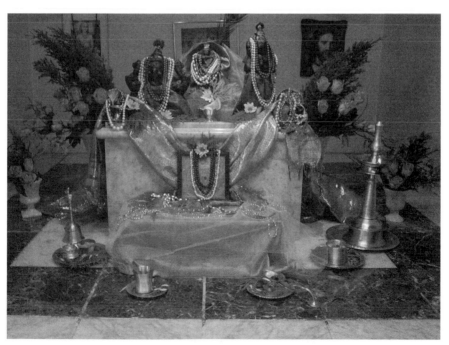

The altars in ashrams often display objects and images that encompass the spiritual focus of the ashram's many visitors. Fresh fruit and flowers are also an important part of decorating the altar.

devoted his life to yoga and is one of the senior disciples of Swami Vishnu. He is a Californian by birth and came of age during the Vietnam era, while he was a student at the University of California at Berkeley. When he talks about the altar, he understands why people are confused. He was not born a yogi or a Hindu, so he knows very well what we want to know.

The temple is quiet after the chanting as he turns toward the altar. The idols and images of gods and gurus are arrayed there in a splendor that seems very exotic in upstate New York. They look as if they had dropped down from another world.

"There are many kinds of idols," he says with a gesture to the altar.

"We create all kinds of idols. Most of the idols in this culture are material idols. These are the kinds of idols they spoke about in the Bible, worshiping gold, worshiping power and position, fame. We create icons for all these things, worshiping sex. The media and advertising are full of idols. The whole culture is based on creating these icons. Money is an idol. An idol can be the dollar bill with a president's picture on it. These are some of the idols of our culture."

He pauses to shift gears. "But idols can be very positive. They can be images that remind us of who we are, not in a sense of being separate, but in a sense of being one, of being divine, of being bliss, of being knowledge, of being love. These idols help us to be caring and compassionate."

He turns again to the altar. "The question is, why do we use these images? It's like when you can have pictures of your children on your desk at work to remind you of your love of your children. The pictures of your kids are symbols that remind you of what is important to you. The same is true of the idols on this altar. They are symbols connecting us to something that is important to us.

"What is important to us?" he asks rhetorically. "Some things we give importance to are leading us toward freedom. They lead us back to knowing who we really are. They lead us back to our Self. Every religion has symbols. Christ is a symbol. The Torah is a symbol. Buddha is a symbol. The symbol focuses the mind and concentrates it.

"In the yoga philosophy everything is spirit, all-pervading consciousness. According to yoga, this realization of the Absolute is the same in all religions. The question is, how do we let go of our identification with the body and the senses? How do we let go of our fears and ambitions? How do we identify with the spirit? Yoga says you can concentrate your mind on religious symbols from any tradition. From there you can explore that aspect of divinity until it expands and includes everything. Swami Vishnu felt that people made the most spiritual progress when they worshiped the symbols they were most familiar with."

Someone asks, "But why are there so many different symbols of God on the altar if any one of them will do?"

"Different people see divinity in different places," says Sri. "The altar is a place of focus. If you can see God in one place, you can see God everywhere. The central focus on this altar is Krishna. Krishna represents God as love, the love that gives meaning to our life, the love that is all-knowledge. Krishna is the indweller of all beings as pure love. Krishna is a symbol that reminds us that God is love and the purpose of life is love. The flute that Krishna plays stands for us. He is making music through us. Krishna leads us from false values and false idols and leads us to the knowledge that all is love."

Again he turns back toward the altar and motions to the image beneath Krishna.

"This is Durga," he adds, "the Divine Mother. She's like Mary. The Divine Mother is also the Mother Earth. The first relationship we have is with the mother. And for many people, identifying with the mother is like identifying with all creation. Durga is both loving and ferocious when it comes to saving us from our lower selves. See, she is riding on a tiger. To her right is someone you are all familiar with, Jesus. He is a symbol of the love of God. On her left is Sankaracharya, a great yogi who founded this order of yoga that we practice. He lived sometime around the eighth century. We practice his *advaita* philosophy that says there is one God. Above him is a picture of Swami Sivananda, one of the great saints of the last century. He really made yoga accessible to the West. He wrote hundreds of books in English. His teaching is to serve, love, give, purify, meditate, realize. He trained many swamis and our founder, Swami Vishnu-Devananda, a master of Hatha Yoga and Raja Yoga. That is his picture on the right."

With Swami Vishnu, he finishes with all the pictures and turns his attention to the white marble altar, about the size of a footlocker, beneath them. The statues on the altar are dressed up in fancy, sequined clothes and festooned with flowers.

Sri points to a teapot-sized image. "On the left of the altar is the elephant-looking statue of Ganesha. If you go to any Hindu temple, you always find Ganesha. He is like the 'Om' spoken before the mantra. He represents pure bliss. By remembering that he is pure bliss—he surmounts all obstacles."

Sri has a thought that makes him smile. "Sometimes Ganesha gives us some obstacles so that we can learn to let go. Obstacles are a way he shows us how to see our limitations and bring us back." Amused at the ways of Ganesha, Sri shows a toothy grin and continues.

"The statue on the right is Hanuman. He is the incarnation of *prana*, or the life force. The main way we experience life is through the mind, and the mind is like a monkey. We all know how hard it is to control the mind, but the way Hanuman controls the mind is through devotion. If you turn your mind toward God, the monkey mind becomes calm. Hanuman is always repeating the name of Ram. He is the embodiment of devotion, of the mind, and of the life force.

"The little statue on the left is the Siva lingam," he says. It looks like an egg in an egg cup sitting in a saucer with a spout on it. There are many

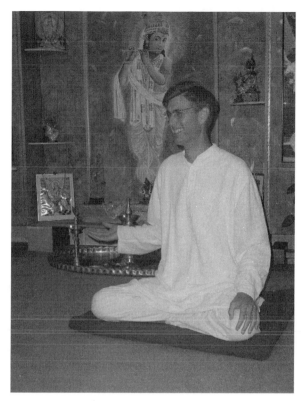

Srinivasan gestures toward the image of Krishna painted behind the altar. He explains that the Hindu gods are different paths to the same truth. There is unity in the seeming diversity of the idols and images.

symbols for Siva. The best known is the *Siva Nataraj,* or Dancing Shiva, the one with six arms dancing in a circle. This Siva lingam is purely abstract, a primordial phallic symbol.

"Siva is a symbol that reminds us of the absolute consciousness in which life is a cosmic dance of creation and destruction. Remember that nothing dies. Everything changes."

The discussion ends with that statement, and *satsang* finishes soon after the final chant, called *Arati:* the waving of the light. We stand and pay homage to all the gods and gurus as one of the devotees who has been trained in the ritual waves a candle before the altar. All the idols mentioned earlier are given this respect, along with many others. As the chant finishes, the candle is carried through the temple so that all can take some of the light for themselves.

The final ritual of *satsang* is *prasad,* food that has been offered to God first and then passed around to all the worshipers. By taking the *prasad* we share food with God. It is always taken with the right hand.

By the time morning *satsang* has ended, you are well prepared for the rest of the day. The ashram day is remarkably well designed, as each activity makes you hungry for what happens next. After almost two hours of sitting, your body has an appetite for exercise. You can't wait for *asana* class. After *satsang,* the ashram staff members stay behind in the temple to discuss what chores must be done that day and who will do them. For the guests, this is teatime, a chance to socialize for about fifteen minutes before the start of the morning *asana* class. You really appreciate having a short break, and these few minutes seem almost giddy. Chanting can get you really high, and the *prasad* is usually sweet. People chatter like birds until the bell rings, announcing that *asana* class is about to begin.

3

Standing on Your Own Head

Yoga without spirituality is mere acrobatics.

—B. K. S. IYENGAR

Asana classes are the backbone of the ashram experience. They hold the day together. The word *asana* means "posture." According to the Yoga *Shastras* there are 840,000 *asana*s, of which eighty-four are considered important. Of these, Swami Vishnu-Devananda considered twelve to be essential. With "so many *asana*s and so little time" in mind, he designed the basic Sivananda class for the maximum physical, mental, and spiritual benefit to students. After taking the month-long Sivananda Teachers Training Course at the ashram in south India, I began to teach classes at the Sivananda Center in Manhattan. Every yoga teacher is a student, too, and we take the same class that we teach. What I have learned about yoga is one part what I was taught and another part what I have learned from within while doing it. The ashram schedule gives me time to explore this intimate terrain from the outside in.

A healthy and flexible spine makes for a healthy and flexible mind. At the ashram, the *asana* practice is one part of the program that makes the other parts work better. They are a ritual that coordinates the body, mind, and breath. As soon as you roll your sticky yoga mat onto the floor, the body knows that it is being cared for, and the mind is calmed.

Practicing *asana*s makes it easier to sit for longer periods of meditation. The *asana*s make it easier to sleep at night. They give you more control over your mind and body. The results cannot be denied, but they do not come all at once. Your legs may still fall asleep and your hips still ache after you have sat cross-legged for an hour, but at least you can do it. *Asana* class is itself a form of meditation.

Hatha is a combination of two Sanskrit words: *ha*, which means "sun," and *tha*, which means "moon." These are the two sides of you that yoga unites. Doing the *asana*s, you become one with your self on a spiritual level. On the physical plane, the *asana*s loosen and lubricate the joints, stretch the muscles and tendons, and enhance the flow of blood and oxygen into the body. They fire up the digestive system. The ashram's healthy vegetarian diet works hand in hand with the practice of Hatha Yoga. The purification of the body and mind goes much faster when you have a proper diet to go along with proper exercise and breathing. Ashram life removes the obstacles to give you everything you need to make real progress.

Dancing with Your Breath

At Sivananda ashrams, attendance is mandatory for both morning and afternoon sessions. Taking two classes makes you feel as if you are truly living yoga. In the morning, you are strong but stiff. In the afternoon, you are not quite so strong but more flexible. Between the two, your practice can only become deeper. You will also have two different teachers in the course of the day. Even though the classes follow the same order of poses, no two classes are alike. They vary according to the teacher. One way to think about *asana* class is that it is a dance. At first you struggle just to learn the steps. Then you learn to put them to music—the breath. When you know the steps and put them to music, you are dancing. Even though the steps are the same and the music is the same, no two people do them in just the same way. Somehow, individuality is heightened. You cannot help being yourself, and your *asana* practice is a reflection of your inner nature.

An experienced instructor can teach you how to dance to the rhythm of your breath, how to lose yourself in the music and go with the flow. The teacher leads, and you follow. At first you feel as if you are stumbling around and stepping on your own toes, but as class follows class a change occurs. A magic moment comes when you are learning how to dance, when you let go and start to move with the music. Suddenly you are in the dance. It happens when you least expect it. This is the moment you have been working toward. The teacher is dancing with the class, too, because dancing is a two-way street. By using intuition to set the tempo and by applying knowledge based on personal practice, the teacher helps you break through from awkwardness to grace. A good dancer can dance with anyone, and a good teacher can teach anyone to dance. You learn fast when you have two teachers a day and four hours of class. Pretty soon you are not looking down at your feet anymore. You are listening to your breath and moving to the music even when you hold the pose in perfect stillness.

You might not understand everything the teacher tells you the first time you hear it. Some of the instructions may seem vague in the beginning, but later they will seem obvious. It helps to keep an open mind and use common sense. Once you start to find your way through your own inner experience, many doubts will subside and vanish. It is said that yoga is not a religion but the science of religion. Testing things to find the truth is the essence of the scientific method. Yoga is a never-ending process. Teachers, too, need to do this in their own practice, and good teachers do. They speak with the authority that comes from personal experience. You can feel this knowledge through your own intuition. Listen to the teacher, and listen to your body. They are both your teachers. They are both your dance partners. Show up on the dance floor ready to have a good time, and you have taken the first step. The more fun you have in class, the faster you will progress, so try to bring a light heart to class with you. Once you are there, all you have to do is pay attention. The results can be surprising. At an ashram, dramatic changes in your *asana* practice can happen much more quickly than you would expect.

Laksmi has been a Sivananda teacher for twenty years. She is co-director with her husband, Srinivasan, of the upstate New York Yoga Ranch. I have taken her classes many times, and I am still mystified by her teaching. Many serious students have told me that she is one of the best teachers they have ever had, and I agree. In her classes I get deeper into the postures with less effort. The two hours seem to go by in twenty minutes. With her help I find a focus that transcends time. She

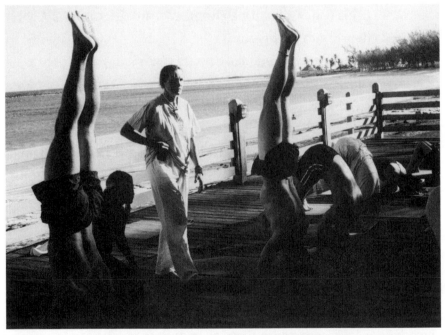

Ashrams have a designated location for daily asana *practice, a serene, quiet place where it is easy for students to focus. Often the classes are conducted outside, where students can stay in touch with nature. Laksmi passes through a portal of head-standing students at the Sivananda Ashram Yoga Retreat on Paradise Island in the Bahamas, as the Atlantic Ocean shimmers in the background.*

is serious and playful, with a self-confidence that comes to a person who has thorough knowledge and long practice. She never preaches when she teaches. Her instructions are simple and direct. They are minimal— yet they are exactly what you need to hear. She seems to know intuitively how students think. She never says too little or too much.

When I ask her how a student can get the most out of a Hatha Yoga class, she says with a pronounced French accent, "Come with an open mind, no preconceived ideas, just let it happen and get into the flow."

"What about beginners when they come to the ashram?" I ask.

"Of course, if someone has never done it before, four hours of class- es can make them quite miserable the next day." She even laughs with a French accent. "Don't write that. But you know what I mean. If they accept the fact that there are things they can't do and just do what they can, they can be happy and have a good experience right away. If they try too hard with a lot of pulling and pushing, that is no good. Sometimes it's better not to have experience. That way the mind is more open."

"Is the same true for people who have a lot of experience?" I ask.

"If people have experience, sometimes they come with an idea of what they expect the class to be," she replies. "Those who come with this attitude don't get as much out of it. The ideas people have about how things should be done causes them to resist—especially if they get something different than what they expect."

When I ask her if there was anything special that she tried to get through to students, she smiles again as if the question were just a lit- tle bit silly. She is lighthearted about yoga. Maybe that is her secret. "Yes, but it's not exactly like that. I just go and teach the class. I want people to feel good, to let go so they can discover what is on the inside. When I teach I just let it happen, like I am an instrument of the teaching. What I try to do is to make the people come out of the class feeling good, or relaxed. When they let go of physical tightness they let go of something else they are holding inside. When people do *asana*s they find something else is there. It's not just that it feels good, but something passes through them. If they just let themselves flow, they can discover that they can do more than they ever thought they could. The teacher is guiding you, and if you don't pull or push you can go far."

Over years of teaching she has seen her focus shift in some ways as meditation has become even more important to her. "It is *you* that comes through when you teach," she says. "I used to be more into the *asana*s for themselves. I liked to do things that were hard, and my classes reflected that. I liked the challenge. Now I look at the *asana* as a tool to feel good and to be able to sit [in meditation]. But when I teach a group of students who are young and healthy and want to do things that are difficult, I will challenge them to keep them entertained. I tell them to just treat it like a game. I say, 'Let's play.'"

A Class Taught by a Master

Since *asana* classes are such an important part of the ashram experience, let's take one together. I will describe a morning class taught by Laksmi at the Sivananda Ashram Yoga Retreat in the Bahamas. The month is January, and the temperature is eighty degrees. The platform is open to the sky, and waves of blue-green water break placidly on a white sandy beach. The sky is clear. The sun has not yet risen above the palm trees. My bottom is sore from sitting cross-legged in the temple for almost two hours at *satsang*. When I arrive, half the class is already lined up flat on their backs on their sticky mats in *savasana*, Corpse Pose. I lie down in my favorite spot under the branches of an old pine. I let myself steep in relaxation as tea is released into water. It's only eight o'clock, but I have been up since after five. This is the time of day when I normally wake up at home. Part of me, the lazy part, wants to go back to bed.

Savasana is considered the most difficult posture to master, but it has many benefits. A great deal of mind control is necessary for completely letting go. It takes a lot of concentration to let go of all the tension in the body and all the thoughts that bubble up.

Once I asked Laksmi which *asana* she would choose if she could have only one, and she answered, "Relaxation. If you can let go totally, in fifteen minutes you can recharge yourself for two hours. Through relaxation you can touch your inner self. When I first started with yoga, it was through relaxation that I felt something different. When you are lying there, something comes through you that changes you. This is the kind of feeling that will teach you to go further. You know yourself how the students come in so tense with the whole world on their shoulders, and they leave relaxed and happy inside and out."

At five minutes after eight she begins the class. "Lie down with your legs about shoulder width apart, arms away from the body, palms facing upward, chin slightly tucked in. Feel where your body is in contact with the floor, and feel the relaxation enter from the soles of your feet, traveling up the legs. We use autosuggestion now. Repeat silently to yourself, 'My legs are relaxing. My legs are completely relaaaxed. My thighs and hips are relaxing. My thighs and hips are completely relaaaxed.'" In this way she goes through the entire body to the top of the head; then she goes through the internal organs. I feel the autosuggestion working as my lower back sinks down, coming into contact with the floor. I listen to the waves lapping the beach. I enter a dreamlike state.

As I lie there thinking about how wonderful life can be, gnats start to buzz around my ear. My mood shifts quickly from transcendence to irritation. I reach up and brush them away. This futile gesture never works, but what else can I do? The gnats always come back. As soon as they are gone I start to dread their inevitable return. When they come back it gets worse. The bravest of the lot has gone exploring in my ear canal. I feel it walking around in there, buzzing and fluttering its wings. I decide to let the gnats do whatever they please and hope they get bored with my ear before I go crazy. But I am not sure that gnats ever get bored.

I try to look at the bright side. At least these particular gnats don't bite. I summon all my mental strength and vow to leave them alone and hope they go away.

During the next five minutes in Corpse Pose, I act like a dead man and don't move, but I would not say that I am relaxed. The gnats are bold. A gnat jamboree is going on in my ear. I have doubts about whether this is a good idea. What if they lay eggs in there? Then I'll be sorry. Just as I am about to go mad, they fly away. I sigh with relief. I know they will come back, but I don't care. I have won the battle for now. I try to beat back the pride I feel, but I cannot.

This titanic struggle has ended, I hope, when Laksmi says, "Now wiggle your fingers and toes, and let the awareness come back into your body. Roll over on your right side and rest for a moment, and then come up and sit up straight in a comfortable cross-legged position for the opening prayer."

When we are all sitting up, she sings a sweet-sounding chant called *Gajananam* to spiritualize the practice. All Sivananda classes start with this chant, which is really a long mantra invoking various deities and asking for their help and protection. This ritual is similar to a football team reciting the Lord's Prayer before the game. The difference is that there is no battle going on here, except with your lower self and maybe the gnats. Yoga *asana*s are rituals, and it helps when you think about them in this way.

Breathing exercises called *pranayama* are performed next. Literally, *pranayama* means controlling the *prana*, or cosmic energy. This *prana*, which pervades the universe, is one of the most important concepts of yoga. We absorb *prana* by breathing, eating, and sunshine, and we store it in our brain and nerve centers. It is intangible, but you see it everywhere. In *Bliss Divine*, Swami Sivananda describes it like this: "It is *Prana* that shines in your eyes. It is through the power of *Prana* the ear hears, the eyes see, the skin feels, the tongue tastes, the nose smells, the brain and the intellect do their functions. The smile of a young lady, the melody in the music, the power in the emphatic words of an orator, the charm in the speech of one's beloved, are all due to *Prana*. Fire burns through *Prana*. Wind blows through *Prana*. Rivers flow through *Prana*."

By doing *pranayama* we store up the *prana*. The first exercise is called *kapalabathi*, which literally means "shining skull" because when you do it you feel as if your skull is actually shining. *Kapalabathi* is also a *kriya*, or cleansing exercise. It clears the nasal passages and gets rid of bronchial congestion by the repeated forcible exhalation of the breath through the nose.

"Sit up straight," says Laksmi, "and prepare yourself for *kapalabathi*."

This is an advanced class, and everyone knows what to do. I sit up and check my posture. Laksmi instructs us to take three deep yogic breaths. In yogic breathing you inhale the air all the way down into the stomach so that the navel moves away from the spine. Then the chest is filled all the way up to the space under the collarbone. When you exhale, the chest is emptied and then the lower lungs.

"Now begin." Laksmi sets the rhythm, repeating, "ONE, two . . . ONE, two . . . ONE, two . . ." With a straight back I vigorously pump the air out of my lungs. I do this forcefully and rhythmically, pushing the air out of the nose and letting it come back in on its own. Having a tissue nearby is a good idea because the nose might run at first. We pump about sixty times, take two yogic breaths, and hold our breath for one minute. One minute is a long retention for the first round, but this is an advanced class. We are free to let go any time we like. *Kapala-bathi* is not a contest to see how long we can hold our breath. As I hold the breath in the lungs I concentrate on the *ajna chakra*, the space between my eyebrows, and hope the gnats don't come back. I try to imagine that energy and light are rising up from the *muladhara chakra* at the base of my spine, up the *shushumna nadi*, which according to yoga is the major energy channel in the middle of the spinal cord. I

concentrate on bringing this energy, which is *prana,* up the spine vertebra by vertebra to the point between my eyebrows.

All the *chakra*s, or energy centers of the astral body, correspond to
nerve plexuses in the physical body. There are seven of them, and they
are located on the *Shushumna nadi.* As the *prana* travels upward and
pierces these *chakras* one by one, higher and higher levels of spiritual
awareness are experienced until the *prana* reaches the highest level at
the crown of the head, the *sahasrara chakra.* In the physical body this
corresponds to the pineal gland. When the energy has moved all the
way to the top, a state of superconsciousness is achieved. In most people
this is a very long road indeed. Another name for this energy is *kundalini
shakti.* To arouse this energy requires a pure heart, mind, and body. The
devotee must be full of devotion, wisdom, and selfless service. Luckily,
this is not an all-or-nothing proposition. If even a little bit of *prana*
moves up the *shushumna,* higher states of consciousness are felt.

We do three sets of *kapalabathi,* and on the third round the breath
retention is two minutes—if we can last that long. There is nothing to
be gained by trying to hold the breath longer than you are able. As in
all Hatha Yoga practices, the wise student will know his or her limits
and work within them. To do this is far better than to incur injury by
pushing too hard, especially since self-knowledge is the key to progress.
I repeat my mantra to help me last the full two minutes. My concentration this day is good. At the finish, I let the air out slowly with control. It takes me a week of ashram living to be able to hold my breath
this long. My skull really does feel as if it is shining.

Next we are led through alternate-nostril breathing, or *analoma viloma.* This exercise is commonly seen in popular depictions of yoga where
the yogi sits in meditation pose and pinches the nose shut with the right
hand. When we breathe normally, one of the nostrils will be partly
blocked and most of the breath will come through the nostril that is
more open. In a healthy person, the breath will go through one nos-

tril for about an hour and fifty minutes and then change to the other side. When we practice *analoma viloma*, we force the breath to change sides by opening and closing the nostrils with the thumb and fingers of the right hand. The practice is easier to demonstrate than to describe, but the gist of it is to inhale on one side to a count of four, pinch off both nostrils for a count of sixteen, exhale on the other side to a count of eight, and then reverse sides and do it over again.

Unluckily for me, the clever gnats are back. I think they have noticed that both my hands are occupied and that in my present condition I am unlikely to swat them. I am tempted mightily to smack myself in the ear to kill them once and for all. The only thing that stops me is the knowledge that there are more where they came from. This time they crawl into both of my ears at once. It sounds as if they are having a big party in stereo. The sensation is that of being tickled maliciously. As I alternate breathing from nostril to nostril they alternate biting from ear to ear. It actually crosses my mind that the sensation is something like sex, only in the wrong place. I am approaching an orgasm of annoyance when they finally get tired of the game and fly away. I am proud as a peacock that I have outlasted them again. Despite knowing that this war of wills between gnats and me has no significance, I see this as a major personal breakthrough. I feel that I have gained a smidgen of self-control. We lie back and rest for a couple of minutes in *savasana* and feel the subtle changes in the body brought on by the practice of *pranayama*. I am more awake and aware, and I have a feeling of lightness in my limbs.

Before the practice of *asana*s proper, we warm the body with the Sun Salutation, or *Surya Namaskar*. In ancient times, people practiced this exercise in the early morning while facing the sun as a form of worship. As a New Yorker on a yoga vacation in the Bahamas in January, I have no problem with this. The sun is just rising above the palm trees as we begin. Laksmi instructs us to stand at the tops of our mats in Mountain Pose, *tadasana*. Mountain Pose is a form of standing meditation. All you really do is stand there, but the difference between *tadasana* and just standing is the difference between doing something consciously and doing it unconsciously. We take a moment to feel our feet holding strong to the floor with the weight equally distributed on the balls of our feet and heels. We imagine that we are as steady as a mountain. This kind of posture is all about having a straight back, being aware of the balance, and letting go of any tension that is not vital to standing tall. We stand in this pose about as long as it just took you to read this description of it. Then the Sun Salutation begins. We follow Laksmi's commands as she sets the tempo, which starts slowly and builds speed as it goes along. The Sun Salutation is a complete exercise in itself, and it is the perfect warm-up for the *asana*s.

There are twelve positions, and each one is coordinated precisely with the breath. First we inhale, and then we begin.

One: On the exhalation, I bring the palms together in prayer position.

Two: On an inhalation, I stretch up with my arms close to my ears, looking up at my hands as I stretch backward.

Three: Exhaling, I bend at the waist and try to get my palms flat on the floor, fingertips in line with toes. I can't get all the way down without bending my knees. If I can't get my palms flat on the floor, it is all right to bend the knees.

Four: Inhaling again, I thrust my right foot back and look up to the sky. My left knee is directly over my left ankle. The right knee rests on the mat, and so does the top of the right foot. This stretches out the hips.

Five: Holding the breath, I thrust the left leg back. Now I am in push-up position.

Six: Exhaling, I lower my knees, chest, and forearms to the mat with my buttocks sticking up in the air.

Seven: Inhaling, I raise my head, using the strength of the back and the arms, and stretch my legs out behind.

Eight: Exhaling, I push up on my arms and lift my buttocks to the sky. My heels are pressing down into the mat. This position is called Downward Dog.

Nine: With an inhalation, I step the right foot forward again between the palms of the hands. Once again I look up to the sky.

Ten: Exhaling, I bring the left foot forward between my hands, which have never moved. I am back in the forward bend.

Eleven: With an inhalation, I raise my hands over my head again.

Twelve: Exhaling, I lower the arms to either side.

That is one Sun Salutation. As a class we will do twelve of these. *Surya Namaskar* is the only aerobic part of a Sivananda yoga class, and it is a complete workout in itself. When we have finished, the back is loose, the breath is regulated, and we have a good sweat. Now all the muscle groups are warmed up, and we are ready to hold the postures with confidence. Laksmi has set a pace that is slow at first, with an increasing tempo as we go along. When we finish, we lower ourselves to the mat and rest for a couple of minutes in *savasana* in preparation for the king of the *asana*s: the Headstand.

When Swami Vishnu said, "I came to America to teach people how to stand on their own heads," he wasn't kidding. The Headstand, or *sirsasana,* has many benefits. It brings oxygen-rich blood to the brain, lets the heart relax, focuses the mind, increases memory, and brings self-confidence. When students learn the Headstand they are very happy. I love to teach it, because it is easier than it looks, and it makes students feel like real yogis.

I turn myself around so that when I come up I will be facing the

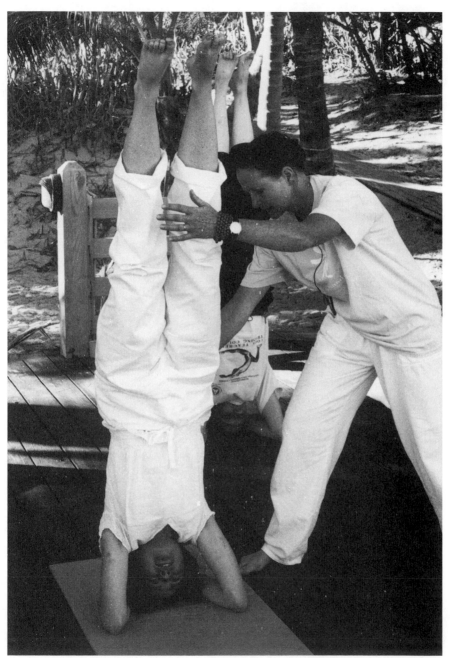

In the headstand, the back should be held as straight as possible with the arms carrying most of the weight. "Close your eyes, push down on your forearms, and pull your shoulders up away from your ears," Laksmi advises.

ocean. Usually, I close my eyes when doing the Headstand, but it is not every day that I can look out to sea while I am upside down. Laksmi tells us to hold the position for five minutes before trying any variations. Seeing the horizon when I am upside down makes me feel as if the whole world has turned upside down, not just me.

While we hold the position, she gives us instructions: "Put very little weight on your head. Support yourself by pushing your arms into the mat. Pull your shoulders up away from your ears. Don't collapse into the posture." As the minutes go by, not collapsing gets harder and harder. Fighting gravity makes my arms tired, and I feel more and more weight shift from my arms to my head. I am sinking downward when a gnat buzzes my ear. Now I couldn't swat it if I wanted to. Irritation brings with it a shot of adrenalin, and I push my arms down fiercely into the mat and lift my head off the platform into the Scorpion Pose. Now I am balanced with all the weight on my forearms. My friend the gnat has brought me a burst of energy. I ignore it as I shift my weight over my elbows and bend myself backward, lowering my feet down toward my head. When the gnat flies away I lower myself back to the mat with control and rest up for the queen of the *asana*s: the Shoulderstand, or *sarvangasana*.

Lying on my back, I lift my legs to make a right angle to my body. Then I bring my hands to my buttocks and lift them off the floor, walking my hands down toward my shoulders until my weight is resting on my shoulders and upper arms. My feet are in the air, and my chest is pushing into my chin. As I get used to the position I work on getting my body as straight as possible. *Sarvangasana* brings a rich supply of blood to the thyroid gland, helping to regulate the metabolism and control body weight. In addition, the Shoulderstand, as an inverted posture, brings many of the same benefits as the Headstand. As I hold myself in the position I close my eyes and try to relax my face.

When you practice *asana*s, it is best to use only those muscle groups that are really necessary to hold you in the position. By controlling the facial muscles, you begin to master all the muscles. By relaxing all the muscles that are not necessary to hold the pose, you are able to stay in the positions for longer periods. You never get the maximum benefit until you can relax and remain perfectly steady.

From Shoulderstand you come into the next posture—the Plow, or *halasana*—by lowering the feet to the floor over the head. If you can get the feet all the way to the floor, you lower your arms behind you and put your palms flat on the floor. Otherwise, continue to support the back. *Halasana* gives an extra stretch to the back of the neck and brings more flexibility to the spine. Done regularly, it removes the signs of aging around the neck and massages the internal organs.

To get into position for the next posture, we raise our legs back up into the Shoulderstand, supporting the back again. Then, one leg at a time, without moving the hands, we bring our legs down and our feet to the floor the other way, making a bridge with our backs. Our navels are pointed up to the sky. This position is called the Bridge, or *setubandhasana*. It reverses the stretch of the Shoulderstand and makes the spine and wrists supple. The liver and spleen are stimulated, enhancing the body's ability to digest fats and regulate the blood sugar.

The counter pose to the Shoulderstand is the Fish Pose, *matsyasana*. To get into it, lie flat on your back with your legs together. Bring your arms under your body, rocking from side to side to get them as close together as possible with your palms face down under the thighs. Bend your elbows, push them into the floor, and use them to lift the chest. Let your head drop back, and rest it on the floor with most of the weight held by the arms. In this position the chest is greatly expanded so large amounts of air can enter the lungs. The Fish Pose increases lung capacity and strengthens the entire back. It should be held for half as long as the Shoulderstand.

Following the Fish Pose is the Forward Bend, or *pashchimotanasana*. In this position, we sit on the floor with our legs together in front of us.

The feet are flexed with the toes curled back toward the face. We reach up to the sky as high as we can and then bend forward, folding at the hips. Our hands take hold of the feet as we use the breath to go deeper and deeper into the posture. With each inhalation we lengthen the spine, and with every exhalation we lower our chest toward the thighs. Laksmi reminds us that this is a position of surrender, so you do not want to be pulling yourself down. Instead, let gravity and the breath do the work for you. In the forward bend, as in all the positions, it is supremely important to breathe. It is the breath that brings us into perfect alignment. When we breathe correctly and continuously, the postures come easily. The benefits of the Forward Bend are best realized when it is held for at least five minutes. The importance of this *asana* is highlighted in the *Hatha Yoga Pradipika*, the most important text on the subject of Hatha Yoga. Its sources are ancient, but it was first written down in the seventeenth century by Yogi Swatmarama. It says, "This most excellent of *asana*s makes the breath flow though the *shushumna,* rouses the gastric fire, makes the loins lean, and removes all diseases."

After the Forward Bend, immediately do a counter stretch called the Inclined Plane. Sit up straight again with your legs together, and put your hands behind you with the palms down. Drop the head back, lift your hips to the sky, and try to get all ten toes on the floor. This is the hard part. The Inclined Plane counters the Forward Bend, increasing blood circulation and strengthening the shoulders, arms, and hips.

The next three *asana*s are back bends. The first and most important of the three is the Cobra, *bhujangasana*. To prepare for it, come into a resting position.

"Now lie on your stomachs and make a pillow with your hands and rest your head to one side with your cheek on your hands," says Laksmi. "Big toes should be touching with the heels falling away to the sides. Scan your body for tension, and if there is any, then focus the breath on that place and breathe into it. Then breathe out, and let the tension go with it.

"Put your forehead on the floor, and point your feet behind you. Turn your thighs inward so that they touch, and put your hands under the shoulders. With an inhalation, use the muscles of the back to bring your head upward, reaching forward with your chin first and then looking up to the sky. Then push down on the hands, and push up. Squeeze your buttocks together to protect the back. Relax your face and breathe." We do this three times with minor variations and then follow it with the Locust Pose, *salabhasana*.

"Now put your chin on the floor and your arms under your body with the elbows close together. Either make a fist or put your palms face down, whatever you like. We will take three deep breaths, and on the third breath push down on the arms and raise your legs as high off the floor as you can. Inhale energy. Exhale fatigue. Inhale strength. Exhale weakness. Inhale, and come up."

The Locust Pose is a strenuous *asana*, but I have learned to love it. It's like hitting yourself on the head with a hammer—it feels so good when you stop. I push down with my arms and bring my legs up slowly by tightening my lower back. It hurts so good. I hold the position as long as I can. Before lowering the legs, I give it one more effort, and my legs feel as if they are levitating upward. Satisfied, I gently lower them to the floor. I make a pillow with my hands and rest my other cheek on them so that I am looking in the opposite direction. I breathe into my lower back and prepare for the final back bend, the Bow, or *dhanurasana*.

The Bow is a combination of the Cobra and the Locust. Once again I put my forehead to the floor, but this time I bend my knees and reach back and grab my ankles, trying not to spread my legs apart too much. Inhaling, I raise my chest and knees off the floor and stretch my arms like a bowstring. In addition to bringing more strength and flexibility to the spine, the Bow gives the digestive organs a massage. It gets rid of constipation, helps people with diabetes, and takes fat off the middle.

The next *asana*, Half Spinal Twist, or *ardha matsyendrasana*, turns the spine laterally, as when you look over your shoulder. First, sit on your heels and drop your buttocks to the floor outside the left knee. Then put your right foot on the floor outside the left knee. Put your right hand on the floor behind your back. Raise your left arm to the sky, and stretch upward. Then take hold of your right knee with your left hand and pull it toward you, looking over the right shoulder. As you inhale try to lift the head higher, and as you exhale turn farther to the right. Hold the position for about a minute, and then reverse everything and look over the left shoulder, turning the back in the opposite direction. The Half Spinal Twist rotates each vertebra, enhancing side-to-side mobility. It tones the nerves and massages the internal organs.

Remember the gnats? They are gone, but thanks to them I have had an outstanding class. Sometimes in the practice of Hatha Yoga I really have a remarkable session. When I managed to control my senses and let the gnats play in my ears and leave on their own accord, I was very proud of myself. You might say that I was as proud as a peacock. There is a pose called the Peacock, *mayurasana*, and I never thought I would be able to do it. My wrists were never flexible enough, and I never had the arm strength to hold the balance. But today was different. I knelt down and put my palms on the floor between my legs with my fingers facing backward. Then I bent my elbows and pressed them into my stomach, lowering my forehead to the floor. Slowly I straightened out my legs and lifted my head off the floor. Now my whole body was off the floor, perfectly straight and parallel to the floor, as I balanced on my hands. I simply could not believe it. Not only was I doing a pose that I never thought I could manage, but it was easy. I managed to hold it ten seconds the first time. Then, to make sure I was not dreaming, I did it again. For the first time I enjoyed the many benefits of this *asana*. It is extremely invigorating. We get more energy in less time from the Peacock than from any other pose. It tones the abdomen, increases the circulation to all the digestive organs, and awakens *kundalini shakti*.

The rest of the class passed as if I were in a dream. I did the Standing Forward Bend, *pada hastasana*, which is much like the seated Forward Bend, and enjoyed the stretch in the spine and a noticeable lightness of being. For the final *asana*, Triangle, I stood up with my feet about three feet apart, raised my left arm up by my ear and bent over to the right, resting my hand on my leg, stretching the entire left side of my body. Then I turned it around and did the other side. *Trikonasana* tones the nerves in the back and opens the hips. I barely remember anything that came after the Peacock.

Finally, it was time for Final Relaxation. I had just finished the best *asana* class of my life. My body was completely happy. I rested on my back in complete bliss. Laksmi took us through the autosuggestion. "A wave of relaxation is entering the body through the soles of the feet. . ." That is the last thing I remember before falling into a deep sleep.

4

Food for Thought

*A kitchen is the best training ground or school for devel-
oping tolerance, endurance, forebearance, mercy, sympa-
thy, love, adaptability, and the spirit of real service for
purifying one's heart and for realizing the oneness of life.
Every aspirant should know how to cook well.*

—SWAMI SIVANANDA

When I did my Teacher Training Course at the Sivananda Yoga Vedanta Dhanwantari Ashram in south India, I was assigned to serve chai every
morning at 7:30 and again in the afternoon at 1:30. Being the chai-
wallah put me at the social center of the ashram twice a day because I
was dispensing a product that just about everybody wanted. We were
all given daily tasks to do as a Karma Yoga, because selfless service is
considered a cornerstone for any aspirant who wishes to build a solid
spiritual practice. Pouring chai could hardly be called work. It was
really more like throwing a tea party. There were much harder duties
such as cleaning toilets, emptying trashcans, and keeping attendance
rolls, but I took some satisfaction in being on time and serving cheer-
fully. Liking my job was pure good luck, and it gave me a peek into
the workings of the ashram's kitchen. It also gave me some insight into
how seriously the role of food and drink is taken.

The chai was made in a large vat in the ashram's kitchen by boiling loose leaves of black tea with water and milk. It was sweetened with jaggery, an unrefined brown sugar. The result was a beige drink that provided a mild caffeine kick and a sugar rush. If the chai was even slightly behind schedule, there would be a clamor. Most of the time all five heavy, one-gallon stainless steel kettles were already filled and waiting for my tea-serving partner, Sally, and me. We would both carry the precious fluid, a teapot in either hand for balance, through a maze of interior passages to the caffeine-deprived crowd that milled around impatiently by the steps in the temple. They waited there full of anticipation. It's funny how quickly habits can be formed. Occasionally the cook was late, and I could watch him make the chai. If the chai was five minutes late, there was one guy who would come down to the kitchen himself to speed things along. I tried not to let this interloper annoy me, but I was not that enlightened. I had developed an attachment to my job. This reminds me of a joke. Why did the Buddha have such a hard time vacuuming his sofa? He didn't have any attachments.

The Care and Feeding of Samskaras

Swami Vishnu-Devananda liked to tell a story to illustrate how the mind becomes enmeshed in habits. When certain thought waves, *vrittis*, become habitual, they create grooves in the mind called *samskara*s in Sanskrit. Swami Vishnu likened these *samskara*s to the grooves in a record. They could also be compared to ruts in a dirt road. Every time a car goes down the road, the rut gets deeper. Pretty soon it's almost impossible for the wheel to go anywhere else except in that groove. Swami Vishnu described a man walking past a bakery. He sees a chocolate éclair in the window and thinks, "That looks good. I think I'll buy that and take it home for dessert." That thought is a *vritti*. If he keeps walking and forgets about the éclair, no pattern is formed. But if he buys it, takes it home, and eats it, a pattern is begun. Let's say he has to walk past that bakery every day. If he starts buying an éclair every day, a *samskara* has been formed.

The concept of the *samskara* is very useful to illustrate how the mind works. *Samskara*s are not all bad. If you were in the habit of getting up every day at 5:30 and meditating, you would be creating a good *samskara*.

I introduce the *samskara*s now because they are easy to understand where food and drink are concerned. If I had known the concept then, I would have been less annoyed at the guy who had to have his chai at exactly 7:35. But I did get some insight into what Swami Sivananda was talking about when he said, "The whole of *Maya* [illusion] is found in the kitchen." The kitchen is very closely watched. The cook didn't seem to mind at all. He was a cheerful, sturdy man who moved with unself-conscious economy during every step of the process, from stirring to straining and pouring. He never seemed to hurry or worry. I always enjoyed a chance to watch him at work. The way he unconsciously ritualized every movement gave me an inkling of how work could turn into worship.

The kitchen had a pleasing simplicity. Getting there was itself a small adventure to the heart—or rather the stomach—of the ashram. It was worthy of a photo essay in *National Geographic*. You took a walk that wound through a cloistered courtyard that led past the laundry, where orange swami robes dried on the line. At the end of the cloister you descended into the kitchen. Along the way you passed potatoes, cabbages, or beets piled against the wall on the floor, waiting to be prepared for the next meal. There was no need for refrigeration. Nothing was frozen, and food was never saved, reheated, and served again. Ashram food is prepared and served with more in mind than just calories, vitamins, and minerals. It is also a source of cosmic energy, or *prana*. This is the same *prana* that we balance, focus, and store up by doing *asana*s and *pranayama*. Mostly it comes from the air we breathe, but it is also found in sunlight and in foods that grow in the sun. For that reason mushrooms, because they grow in the dark, are not considered to have any *prana* in them, and they are not used at Sivananda ashrams.

The first time I saw the kitchen there, I wondered where the stove was. Instead of the stove I expected, steel rings were suspended over the floor on steel legs, and big heavy-duty gas burners stuck up in the middle under them. Great stew pots sat on the rings. Since it never got cold there, the kitchen was screened like a porch, and the breeze was free to blow through, so you got no kitchen smell. The peeling and paring of vegetables was done outside by assistants wearing saris. Some of the best meals I ever ate came out of that simple kitchen. I think Swami Sivananda would have been pleased. That cook was a great Karma yogi. Complaints about the food were rare. At the end of the Teacher Training Course, the cook and the whole kitchen staff got a rousing cheer of approval from the grateful students.

A great feast was prepared for the graduation celebration. We also had a feast in honor of Swami Vishnu's *Mahasamadhi* day. When a great saint leaves the body, it is not seen as a cause for sadness, but for celebration. A person who has become enlightened in his or her lifetime is called a *jivanmukta*. Such a person is said not to die as a normal person does. His or her passing from this realm is considered a release from the endless cycle of birth and death, and the passing is celebrated with a feast. At an ashram feast the food is served on banana leaves instead of on the sectioned stainless steel plates used for any other meal. The festive banana leaves make it look like a party. Not only is the food more beautiful in contrast to the bright green leaves, it is also said to be more nutritious because nutrients from the fresh leaves are absorbed by the food that is served on them.

Tasting Food by Touch

Knives, forks, and spoons are not used at the Indian ashram. Instead, meals are eaten with the fingers of the right hand. Nothing needs to be cut with a knife. The axiom that food is first tasted with the eyes is both familiar and true, but there is an additional sense, touch, which is introduced when you eat with your fingers. After a couple of days you get used to it, and it seems perfectly natural—actually desirable. The tips of the fingers are very sensitive, and they tell you a lot about the texture and temperature of what you are putting in your mouth. They create a sense of anticipation.

Eating with your fingers brings an extra delight to the act of eating. At first you feel like a baby playing with your food. After a month, utensils seem strange. There was a German woman who insisted on using her very own spoon, and I felt sorry for her because I enjoyed so much eating with my fingers. We learned to eat with our hands by watching the Indians herding the food around their plates, mixing up the dishes with their fingers. There was an art to it that I never really learned. I could get the food from the plate to my mouth, but not gracefully. Still, I loved to stick my fingers into the rice and mix it up with the vegetable stew of tomatoes and okra (called ladyfingers in India). Vegetable stews were a major staple, as was basmati rice. I worked them around until I had a paste that would stick together well enough not to slip between my fingers on the way to my mouth. Only the Indians could manage this gracefully. My right hand would be covered with food by the end of the meal. There were no napkins, and licking the fingers was considered impolite. Even so, it was fun.

The morning meal was served at ten after the *asana* class, and it was the main meal of the day. In the evening we were subtly discouraged from overeating because there was less variety and fewer dishes. This is done by design, so that the evening meditation would not be disturbed by overloaded stomachs.

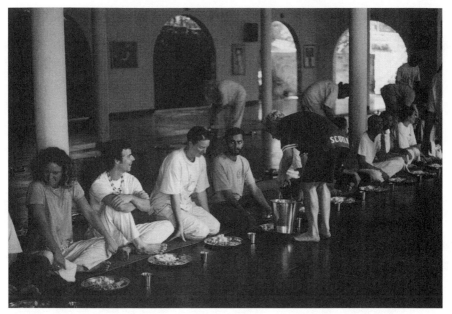

*Meals are taken sitting cross-legged on reed mats. The servers carry the food in pol-
ished stainless steel buckets. The food is eaten using only the right hand. Eating
with your hand is awkward at first and hard to do without making a mess, but by
touching the food you get to know it better.*

At all meals, we sat cross-legged in long lines on mats that were rolled
out on the floor of black marble tile. When I arrived, an empty plate was
waiting. I took a seat and waited for it to be filled by servers who carried shiny stainless steel buckets full of stews or dal (lentils), big bowls
of rice, covered dishes of chowpattis (pancakes) or papadams (big crispy
fried crackers), chopped green beans, sautéed cabbage, boiled potatoes,
beets, tapioca, and the occasional fruit salad. We never served ourselves.
The servers ladled it out. The tapioca was not in the form of pudding;
rather, it was used as a starch, like potatoes. We could have all we wanted, and the servers continued to dole out dishes for the entire time of the
meal. Usually the last thing to be served was thick, almost yogurtlike
buttermilk, which we could drink or mix up with the food. This made
a fine mess. The buttermilk, flavored with herbs and chilies, was sour and

piquant. Coconut was a secret ingredient in many dishes, especially rice, and hidden in many places where it might not be expected. The ashram was in the heart of Kerala, which means land of coconuts, and the coconut palm was as ubiquitous there as corn is in Iowa.

Serving was done by students and staff members as their Karma Yoga. They did not eat until after everyone else had been served. After the meal, we scraped the remains from our plates into a bucket and lined up at a long trough that was studded with spigots. There we washed the plates with a gritty gray soap paste and scrubbed them with the brown fiber from the husk of a coconut. The trough drained into a pipe that poured out on the side of the hill about twenty yards away, where crows would fight over the crumbs of food that washed out. Nothing went to waste.

Ancient Rules for Proper Diet

Ashram meals are prepared using the principles of Ayurveda, literally translated as the "science of life." Ayurveda is said to have been practiced continuously in India for five thousand years, as a healing art that is concerned as much with maintaining health as with curing disease. It takes the whole person into consideration: body, mind, and spirit. One of Ayurveda's most important tools is the regulation of the diet. Because we are what we eat, the choice of foods and how they are prepared cannot be overestimated by one who hopes to make progress in yoga. The yogic diet is vegetarian for both spiritual and material reasons. On the spiritual level, flesh is avoided is because it requires the killing of animals, and *ahimsa,* or noninjury, is a basic principle for living the spiritual life. On the physical level, meat (especially beef) is saturated with fat and pumped full of toxins, growth hormones, and antibiotics. So much has been said and written about this that there is no purpose in going further into it here, but it has to be mentioned.

All foods can be categorized according to the three *gunas,* or cosmic qualities. According to yoga, everything in nature is composed of these three *gunas,* called s*attwa, rajas,* and *tamas.* The ideal yogic diet is *sattwic,* which means pure and balanced. A *sattwic* diet is designed to raise consciousness and enhance the practice of yoga by promoting mental harmony. One way to understand what goes into a *sattwic* diet is by describing what is not *sattwic:* meat and fish, anything canned or processed or raised using chemical fertilizers and pesticides, and any food that is overcooked or reheated. The quality of *sattwa* can also be used to describe people and places. A *sattwic* person is someone who is balanced, cheerful, and loving. In nature, a *sattwic* place is neither too hot nor too cold. It has fresh air and lots of sunlight. It is natural and unspoiled. An ashram in the mountains is *sattwic.* White and yellow are *sattwic* colors. Before going into what a *sattwic* diet is, it would be useful to look at the other two *gunas* and how they relate to food.

The second *guna* is *rajas,* and it is characterized by agitation. *Rajasic* food excites the passions and makes the mind race. Meditation is difficult with this kind of diet, which consists of food that is too spicy, salty, or sour. Garlic, onions, chilies, pickles, and vinegar are said to be *rajasic;* so are coffee and alcohol. New York City is probably the world capital of *rajas.* The modern world runs on *rajas.* When you "eat and run" you are being *rajasic.* This quality describes people who are very active, irritable, sensual, and passionate. *Rajas* is not necessarily bad. It is characterized by movement. Red is a *rajasic* color. *Rajasic* people get things done, so they are good to have around. If you owned a company, you would like to have a lot of *rajasic* people on the payroll, as they are good workers. The downside is that they can be fanatical and intolerant. They do not like to admit they are wrong.

Whenever I tell people that onions and garlic are not a part of the ashram diet, they are shocked. They usually say something like, "What, no garlic? Garlic is one of the healthiest foods you can eat! It gets rid of all kinds of toxins and purifies the blood. What's wrong with onions? Onions are good for you. I can't imagine being a vegetarian and not eating onions and garlic. They give the food flavor." I can sympathize with that response because I love onions and garlic as much as anyone. They are left out of the diet not because they are bad for your health but because they are *rajasic* and are said to excite the mind, and that kind of stimulation makes it harder to meditate.

From a yogic standpoint, the least desirable of the three *guna*s is *tamas*. This quality describes food that is stale, artificial, rancid, or greasy. Meat and fish are considered to be *tamasic,* and so are canned foods. Overeating is also *tamasic,* especially if the food is fatty or oily, or made of refined sugar or white flour. A *tamasic* person is lazy and dull, and tends to sleep too much. You would not want to have a *tamasic* person work for you. A sink full of dirty dishes is *tamasic.* Narcotics and marijuana are considered to be *tamasic.* Inertia and apathy are its characteristics, and its color is black.

These three *guna*s, or qualities, are present in all things in different combinations. Even a saint is not perfect all the time. A saint can get angry, and anger is a *rajasic* state of mind. Swami Vishnu was the first to admit that he had a temper. All three *guna*s are present in all people. The difference is in which predominates, and most people are somewhere in the middle. *Sattwa* is the preferred state because it is there that one has the kind of balance needed to discover the real Self, or *Atman* (soul). A very *sattwic* person is rare. We need some *rajas* to get along in the world and accomplish our goals. The problem with *rajas* is its tendency to encourage burnout. We work so hard, so passionately, that we collapse into *tamas.* In the *Bhagavad Gita* the three *guna*s are described this way:

> That which is like poison at first, but in the end like nectar—that happiness is declared to be Sattwic, born of the purity of one's own mind due to Self-realization.

That happiness which arises from the contact of the sense organs with the objects, which is at first like nectar and in the end like poison—that is declared to be *Rajasic.*

That happiness which at first as well as in the sequel deludes the self, and which arises out of sleep, indolence and heedlessness—that is declared to be *Tamasic.*

The Six Essential Tastes

The practice of yoga requires a *sattwic* diet, one that is balanced. Ayurveda uses a formula based on six tastes to balance the diet. The six tastes are sweet, salty, sour, pungent, bitter, and astringent. They should all be present in every meal to ensure that the digestive fire, *agni,* is stimulated and the mind is harmonized. The principle is called *mitahara,* or everything in moderation.

Toward the end of the Teachers Training Course, Dr. S. K. Kamlesh gave a talk at the ashram on how to use the six tastes to create a balanced meal. Dr. Kamlesh is the son of an Ayurvedic doctor who had treated India's prime minister, Jawaharlal Nehru during his life, has served as the president of the International Society of Ayurveda, and comes from a long line of Ayurvedic doctors. He has a balanced, unflappable air. He is neither tall nor short, fat nor thin; he has a smooth, light-brown complexion; a quick smile; and a glowing countenance. To me, he looked like a good advertisement for the diet he described.

According to Dr. Kamlesh, the first taste is sweet, and it is provided by carbohydrates. Sweet includes potatoes, yams, and grains such as rice and wheat. These should account for at least fifty percent of the meal. Sour comes next. Yogurt is in the sour group. Citrus fruits are also sour, and half an orange, lemon, or lime can be included in a meal. It should be added toward the end of cooking to keep the vitamins from being lost. Pungent foods help the body burn calories, and they aid digestion. These are chilies, ginger, clove, cinnamon, nutmeg, and cumin. Bitter-tasting foods purify and clean the system. Dark green leafy vegetables are good sources of the bitter taste; dandelion, spinach, chard, kale, and collards are some examples. Fennel and bitter melon are also sources of this taste. These are good for avoiding constipation. Dr. Kamlesh said that twenty to thirty grams a day of bitter greens is a good amount. The foods that are considered to be astringent are proteins such as lentils, beans, dal, and tofu. These should be seasoned with fresh ginger, fresh coriander, cumin, and curry. Nuts are also astringent. Dr. Kamlesh said that twenty to thirty percent of the diet should be from the astringent category. The final taste is salty. Salt, according to Dr. Kamlesh, is good for mental power but should be used in moderation. In addition to the six tastes, some oil should also be used in cooking. His favorite was extra virgin olive oil. Canola oil is also good because it can take more heat than olive oil before burning.

The first ashram I ever visited was the Yoga Ranch in upstate New York, and I liked the food but found it too bland at first. The spicier stuff served in India was tastier to me. Perhaps my palate was a bit jaded. Before I got into yoga I was a big fan of hot food. I still like it but try to tone it down now so that I can calm my mind for meditation. As a *rajasic* person, I like hot, spicy food. During the first couple of days at the ashram, my taste buds were not satisfied, but that went away. As my mind unwound I needed less stimulating food. After a while, less was experienced as more. I first began to notice this process at work while eating. After two or three days I felt my sense of taste becoming subtler as my mind became calmer.

Our surroundings and the company we keep at the meal are important, too. In his excellent book *Ayurveda and the Mind*, Dr. David Frawley says, "We are not only what we eat, but whom we eat with, as well as where we eat."

Now You're Cooking with God

Blessing the food is a part of this process. Food is symbolically offered to God first. Before we eat a meal at the ashram at the Yoga Ranch, we stand in a circle, hold hands, and chant the *Maha Mantra*, which means "Great Mantra." It goes, "Hare Raama, Hare Raama, Raama Raama, Hare Hare, Hare Krishna, Hare Krishna, Krishna Krishna, Hare Hare." This mantra is always chanted in its entirety and is never broken. It is said to bring purity to the heart and mind and to be the most powerful mantra in our age. After the blessing, we are free to dig in.

The kitchen at the Ranch has the well-worn patina that comes from constant use and thorough cleaning after every meal. In his book *Practice of Karma Yoga*, Swami Sivananda says, "If an ashram is not properly conducted the kitchen becomes a fighting center. The whole of *Maya* [illusion] is in the kitchen. Aspirants begin to fight there. One aspirant

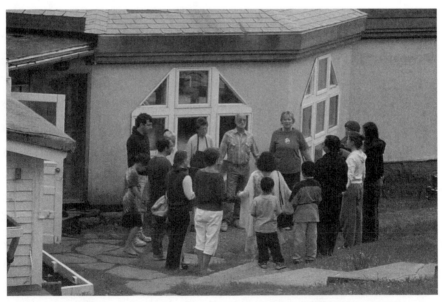

Before every meal the food is blessed by the cooks, ashram staff, and guests. Here everyone clasps hands, forming a circle, and sings the Maha Mantra, "Hare Raama, Hare Raama, Raama Raama, Hare Hare, Hare Krishna, Hare Krishna, Krishna Krishna, Hare Hare." This famous mantra is considered especially powerful.

says, 'I did not get any ghee, or vegetables today.' Another aspirant says: 'The dal soup was very watery.' . . . But if there is a really developed Karma yogi to train the young students, the real Advaita Vedanta [philosophy that God is in everything] begins in the kitchen of an ashram."

I got a firsthand experience in the truth of that recently when I assisted one of the senior staff members in the kitchen at the Yoga Ranch. She is modest and asked that I not use her name, but I can describe her as a devoted, enthusiastic aspirant in her late twenties, who has cooked in ashrams in the United States, Europe, and the United Kingdom.

Preparations for brunch began at eight at the conclusion of the morning meeting of the staff presided over by Srinivasan. The kitchen was clean from the night before, as always. The kitchen cleanup was a full-court press after every meal, and the cooks washed up as they went along. I washed my hands and waited to be told what to do. It was a Friday morning, and the group was small. This would be a good way for me to break in. There were seven staff members and only three guests. The menu was lemon rice, potato suvji, spinach raita, herbed yellow mung dal chelas, and dal soup. There were more kinds of dal than I had ever imagined. The first order of business was to get the potatoes ready for the suvji and the spinach for the raita. While I peeled potatoes, the head chef picked her way through the baby spinach, taking out any wilted leaves and washing the rest. As we stood at the stainless-steel–topped island in the middle of the kitchen, she sang one of the chants from the *kirtan* that had just ended. Few things in this world please me more than to hear a woman singing in the kitchen, but I did not say this. I just soaked it in and did what she told me to do.

Preparing food for a gang of people is a production that has to be well organized so that it's all done by ten o'clock. The chef put a big pot on the eight-burner Vulcan range to steam the spinach after showing me the right-sized chunks into which to cut the potatoes. They were about one-inch cubes and needed to be as uniform as possible so they would take the same time to cook. When I had finished cutting them up, she put a wok on the stove, heated it up, and added some canola oil. After the canola oil was good and hot, she shook some coriander seed, mustard seed, cumin seed, fenugreek seed, and turmeric powder into the hot oil and waited for some of the seeds to pop like popcorn. She was not much for measuring and seemed to know the right amount by feel.

"You know the heat is right when the seeds start to pop," she said. "That is when they release the flavor."

This frying of spices, called making a *chonk*, is done a lot in Indian cooking. The aroma is pungent and delicious and makes you hungry. When the spices were done she added the potatoes, a can of crushed tomatoes, and some water. Canned food is not the most desirable. Fresh tomatoes would have been better, but decent fresh tomatoes cost a fortune in the middle of winter, so the compromise was made.

"Every meal has to have something special, at least one thing," said the singing chef to me as she prepared the batter for the chelas. The chelas are like crepes except that the batter is made mostly of split yellow mung beans that have been soaked overnight. They are pureed in a blender with a little flour to hold the puree together, a dash of baking powder, and enough turmeric to turn the whole batch a bright yellow. If we had had some fresh cilantro, she would have added that too, but we didn't. The batter was then put aside, and attention was turned to the dal soup, which was put on the burner. More frying had to be done to the spices that went into the lemon basmati rice, already steaming on the stove. I juiced a couple of lemons, which she added toward the end of the rice's cooking time along with the spices. Meanwhile I washed the romaine lettuce and broke it into pieces by hand. Had I cut the lettuce with a knife, it would have wilted faster. The chef made a dressing of tahini, lemon juice, and soy sauce with black pepper, and now we were closing in on the finish line.

The chelas were the last dish to be cooked, and she let me do them after showing me how. The trick was to pour the batter from the ladle in a clockwise spiral and use the bottom of the ladle at the same time to spread the batter evenly. This was easier said than done. It looked effortless when she did it, and a perfect thin pancake with the hint of a spiral showing through was the result. The well-seasoned griddle did not need much oil, but after two batches the chelas started to stick. I was in too big a hurry to grease the griddle, and I paid the price. I struggled to make them perfect like hers, but I had to patch and fill a bit so that I would have a pancake and not a spiral string. Still, they were pretty. She added the yogurt to the steamed spinach, and we were done. I looked at the clock and saw that the time was 9:55. Two hours had flown by while we prepared the brunch, and now I had a taste of what it took to feed an ashram. Even though I had played a supporting role, I could not help but feel some pride of authorship, and during the meal I watched closely to see how well the meal was received. Nobody complained; they seemed to be too busy eating to say much.

5

Free Time at the Ashram

A life of discipline is nectar; it is filled with joy.
                                        —BABA MUKTANANDA

The hours between twelve and four at the ashram are called free time, but they are well earned, well deserved, and necessary. Free time at the ashram is just as delicious as lying on your back in Relaxation Pose, *savasana*, at the end of class—and just as important. The chance to relax and just *be* comes at just the right moment. Your body and mind need down-time to drink in the effects of nonstop yoga. If you don't take time out, the yoga starts to feel too much like work. Relaxation is built into the schedule as part of the practice. It feels like a reward for time well spent, a vacation within a vacation. Now you have four hours to do what you please. You can even go back to your room and collapse on the bed without the slightest pang of guilt.

When noon rolls around, your spirit will be elevated and light from meditation. Your heart will be open and free from chanting. Your mind will be focused and engaged by Vedanta. Your body will be relaxed and energized by *asana* practice. Your digestive system will be happily assimilating the vegetarian brunch. And your conscience will be clear from helping with the chores that make the ashram work by doing an hour of selfless service, Karma Yoga. You will be so righteous that you might not recognize yourself. To be more exact, you will recognize a self that you would like to see more often. Free time makes me feel like a school kid when the bell rings for recess.

Touring the Temples

The Sivananda Ashram Guest Handbook lists "walks in the woods, study, workshops, swimming, sauna, meditation, etc." as suitable activities for free time. If you are a first-time visitor, you are offered an optional orientation walk on Saturdays that goes over hill and dale, covering all seventy-seven acres of the property. If you arrive on Friday night, the urge to go straight to your room for a nap on Saturday after doing your Karma Yoga will be strong. The first morning at the ashram is intense. The muscles are stretched out from *asanas*, and your hips may be sore from sitting in meditation pose. I know that mine were at first. Breathing fresh mountain air makes you hungry, and a full stomach makes you sleepy, even if you are used to getting up at 5:30. Take the walk first, and you will still have time for a nap. By taking the tour, you will feel more at home and will know your way around. The tour will give you a chance to meet the other first-time visitors, and you can compare notes.

The group forms at 12:15 outside the temple and heads directly up the hill between the two largest buildings on the compound. The building to the left is called *Kailash,* and it has a large hall on the first floor where *satsang,* special programs, and Hatha Yoga classes are held whenever there are too many people to fit in the temple. In its earlier incarnation it was a banquet hall with a stage at one end. The other building is called *Ananda Kutir,* or Abode of Bliss Absolute. That is where you will probably be staying.

If you are lucky, you will hear some stories about Swami Vishnu-Devananda along the way. He was quite a character. In the foyer of

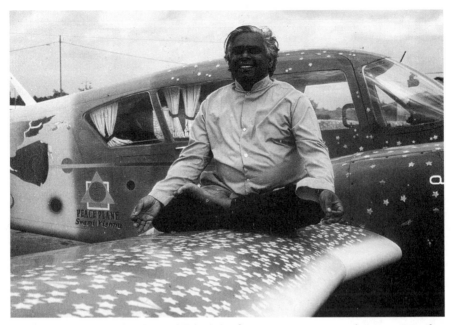

Swami Vishnu-Devananda established the first permanent yoga ashrams in North America. He was daring in his peace missions. His twin-engine Piper Aztec took him on peace missions over northern Ireland and Egypt.

Kailash you will see an unusual shrine—an ultralight para-glider exactly like the one that Swami Vishnu flew over the Berlin Wall at the height of the Cold War on one of his daring peace missions. His nickname was the Flying Swami, and stories of his derring-do are an ashram staple. His twin-engine Piper Aztec plane took him to hot spots all over the world. Part of his life's work was the breaking down of barriers between cultures and religions, and he was a master at manipulating the media with bold stunts to make his point. One of his adventures was a flight over Belfast, Northern Ireland, with the actor Peter Sellers in a bid to cool off sectarian violence. Another was a highly unauthorized mission that took him from Israel over the Suez Canal into Egypt. The Egyptian authorities were not amused when he bombed them with carnations. They sent a fighter plane after him. When he refused their orders to land, the Egyptian pilot blasted him with jet-engine exhaust, nearly knocking him out of the sky. He was forced to land in Cairo, jailed for a short period, and released. The Egyptian authorities really did not know what to make of this fearless swami and his wild-looking plane with its 1970s' Peter Max paint job.

At the top of the hill, the highest point of the ashram's property, stands the Shiva Temple. From its vantage in the middle of a grassy meadow, the view extends for miles in every direction with long blue ridges in the distance. The Shiva Temple is more a shrine than a temple in the Western sense. It serves as a focal point on the property and points to the sky like a lightning rod for Shiva energy. Surrounded by a low block wall, the rustic temple is built of natural wood and looks like a large sentry box. Inside the temple is an altar with small statues of Shiva and other gods standing guard. Daily *puja* is performed there, and an oil lamp is kept lit. There is room to meditate around the altar, and the atmosphere is *sattwic* and mysterious, as befits Shiva, the destroyer of the lower nature. There are two plaques on the wall inscribed with verses from the *Bhagavad Gita*. One says, "For one who sees Me everywhere and everything in Me, I am never lost, nor is he ever lost to Me." The other says, "But those who worship Me with devotion, meditating on My transcendental form, to them I carry what they lack and preserve what they have." The atmosphere inside is solemn and simple. When you sit alone in there, the silence and *sattwa* are palpable.

From the highest point on the ashram, the walk proceeds along a winding path to the lowest point by way of a well-marked trail that takes you down the hill through a hardwood second-growth forest crossed by stone walls built long ago, when this was all pasture. The hill slopes gently downward until the ground levels off again at the bottom, where you enter a stand of cedar. There your footsteps become silent as you tread over the fallen needles instead of crunching leaves. The cedar forest has a hushed, enchanted quality that never fails to surprise me. It is so quiet that you can hear yourself think. Boots are a good idea because rivulets and springs gush forth in the low area, where a gurgling creek follows a rocky bed. Past the cedar forest the path opens again, and you come upon a temple dedicated to the Mother Goddess, Durga. The tiny Durga Temple is built over a concrete pool filled with water and is reached by crossing over a wooden bridge. A sign instructs you to take off your shoes before walking on the bridge. Swami Vishnu used to say that yoga begins when you take off your shoes before entering the temple. Only one person at a time can fit inside Durga's charming temple for sitting meditation. There is no room even to stand. Her temple is like a womb that you can enter only on your knees. When you are in there you feel protected as only the Divine Mother can protect you. The feminine power of this shrine to the Divine Mother situated at the

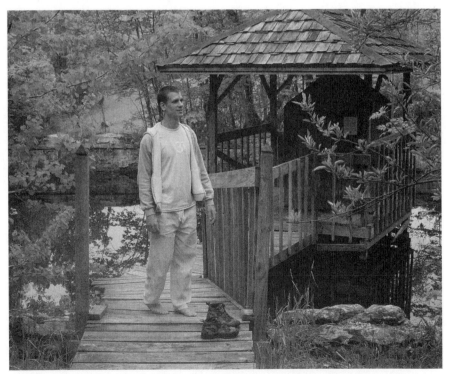

A quiet walk and a visit to a temple is a relaxing way to spend free time while on retreat at yoga ashram.

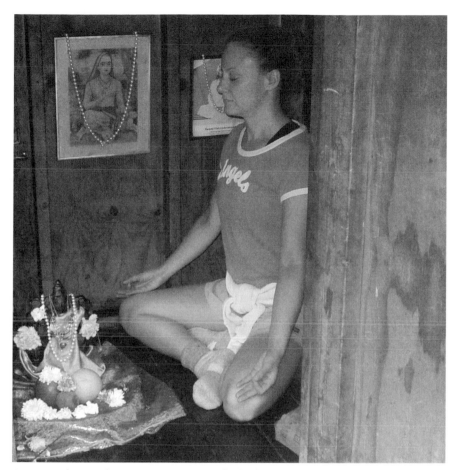

At yoga ashrams there are opportunities for both group and personal devotional rituals. In the Durga temple at the Yoga Ranch, there is only room for one person to enter at a time, which makes it ideal for personal meditation.

lowest, most southern part of the ashram property is said to balance the masculine Shiva energy at the highest point to the north. This balance of powers is said to bring peace to the ashram and to those who go there.

Following along the path, you leave the woods behind and arrive at the cow pasture. In the field are five fortunate bovine creatures. The bull is called Arjuna, and his wife (so to speak) is Padma. They have a daughter, Mookambika (not a joke). And in case you have ever doubted the intelligence of cows, there is one named Prema who ran away from home (a nearby farm) and refused to go back. She made such a fuss about it that the farmer, a kind-hearted man, sold her to the ashram at half price. These four, along with another called Kumakshi, are well cared for, as befits their divine status. When you trespass on their turf, they regard you with benign indifference. Even the bull doesn't have a problem with visitors. As a city dweller I don't have much chance to get up close and personal with cattle, so I make it a point to pet them when I take a walk. I like the way that nothing fazes them. They are living lessons in the art of contentment, *santosha.* This is one of the virtues yogis cultivate in the path of Raja Yoga.

Having treaded carefully through their domain, avoiding the ubiquitous cow pies, you arrive at the entrance to the ashram. Beside the driveway stands a 1970s vintage sign welcoming visitors to the Sivananda Ashram Yoga Ranch Colony. That is the official name. The style of the sign is disarmingly kitsch, but its message is pure Sivananda. Under the smiling visages of Swami Sivananda and Swami Vishnu-Devananda and the symbol for "Om" are words describing the central mission of the ashram in no uncertain terms: "Health Is Wealth. Peace of Mind Is Happiness. Yoga Shows the Way. Serve. Love. Give. Purify. Meditate. Realize." As you contemplate these simple truths that are so hard to put into practice, you leave the cow pasture through a gate that brings you back to the driveway. You turn up the hill and follow the gravel road, and you are soon back where you started.

Working Up a Sweat

The orientation walk puts the Yoga Ranch in perspective. As one of America's first ashrams, it possesses the sincere quality of a pioneering effort. There is nothing at all slick or overdone about this ashram. The buildings sit lightly in the landscape as though they had grown out of it. The atmosphere is down-to-earth and unpretentious. You can see how it took shape and grew organically, one piece at a time. Even Swami Vishnu-Devananda lived in a trailer on the property when he was alive. One of his many mottoes was "Plain living and high thinking." The absence of luxury is itself a luxury.

Across the driveway from the temple is an organic garden and greenhouse complex where some of the vegetables served at the ashram are grown. A gentle, taciturn Irishman named Paul is the head gardener, and he has lived there for about twenty years. He sees to it that all suitable kitchen scraps are composted and that nothing is wasted. His greenhouse is an island of serenity in a sea of calm. A little farther along is an old barn, built into the side of the hill, which serves as storage for the tractors and recyclables. In warm weather, *asana* classes are often held outside there. Down the hill is the sauna, and below that is the swimming pond. Beside the pond are a teepee and the low dome framework of saplings that are used for Native American sweat lodge ceremonies.

The first time I went to the Yoga Ranch, it was on a sweat lodge weekend. I had heard a lot of sweat lodge stories and was anxious to try the experience. Native American traditions are celebrated regularly with special programs. Sometimes they are just on weekends, but weeklong workshops are also held, led by ceremonialists from the Mi'kmag and Mietis/Illinois nations. You can steep yourself in Native American culture with practical lessons of living at peace with the earth, songs, drumming, sunrise ceremonies, forest walks for learning about edible and medicinal herbs, and sweat lodges.

That night of my first sweat lodge experience at the ashram, a great bonfire turned dozens of boulders orange hot under the night sky while more than thirty of us stripped down to shorts and bathing suits and crawled silently inside the round hut made of bent saplings and covered with blankets. It was pitch black and tightly packed with people inside. The air was fragrant from the freshly cut cedar branches that lined the floor. We crowded around a shallow circular pit as the stones were introduced. The heat built slowly as the glowing stones were piled in the shallow pit in the center of the lodge. The stones, the only source of light, had a mesmerizing beauty. We were led in chants to the south and west, north and east. For each direction, more stones were piled. First herbs were sprinkled on the stones, then they were doused with water as we were led in chants. I watched the stones turn from orange to a dull red as buckets of sweat poured out of me. An eagle feather was passed from hand to hand, and everyone there offered a prayer when his or her turn came to hold the feather. When I emerged after about two hours I felt reborn. We stood in a circle holding hands for a final prayer, and then those who wanted to cool off in the pond waded in. Every time I see that lovely frame of saplings I think of that night.

If you don't stop during your walk, the circuit around the Ranch takes about thirty minutes to complete. Whenever I am at the ashram I take this walk almost every day. The distance is long enough for me to feel as if I have stretched my legs and communed with nature without its being a major project. I like to think of it as a mini-*yatra*, or pilgrimage to a sacred place. By calling this little stroll a *yatra* I am making a mild joke to myself, because in India a *yatra* can be a grueling expedition such as a hike to the top of Mount Kailas in the Himalayas. Even so, the idea is the same: to go to a sacred place. The temples to Shiva and Durga are sacred and make fine destinations. If this were a real *yatra*, I would miss the *asana* class at four. Depending on the time of year and the weather, I sometimes carry a pair of binoculars and a bird book. Thanks to the surprising diversity of habitats on the ashram property, bird watching is a satisfying pastime. To see a golden eagle soaring majestically, chickadees flitting nervously, and bluebirds that are singing melodically on the same walk makes me feel the presence of God in flight, as if the birds were messengers. The view through the glasses is another form of meditation.

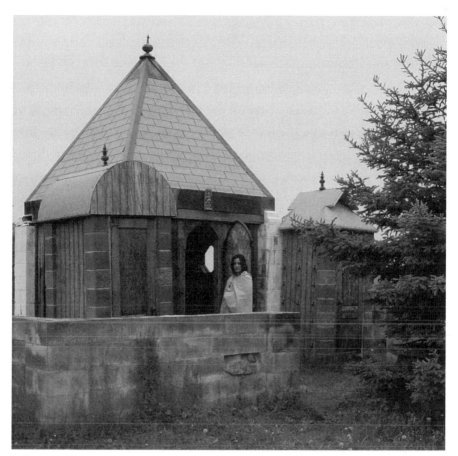

Ashrams offer many opportunities to get away from it all for deep meditation. This rustic temple to Shiva stands in the middle of a grassy meadow on the highest point of the Yoga Ranch ashram's property, a perfect place to dive into silence.

One purpose of ashram life is to spiritualize all you do and see. After a few days your heart starts to open up a little, and so do your eyes and ears. You begin to see nature as the subtle play of God. There is a herd of deer that frolics around the Shiva Temple in the early morning and glides past the Durga Temple in the evening. The rhythms of nature are reflected in the rituals of worship so faithfully that every act has divine potential. After a week at the ashram, barriers start breaking down between you and everything else. This union is what yoga is all about.

No News Is Good News

Newspapers are scarce at the ashram, but they are not banned. Having worked at the *New York Post* for twenty years, I am more than happy not to have newspapers around. When I was news editor there, I would arrive at the office and find a stack of papers and magazines six inches high waiting for me every day, and I had to know what was in them. Don't imagine that I read them all. Editors at newspapers have their own way of speed-reading that is very different from that used by civilians. It's more like osmosis than actual reading. At the ashram, reading the paper feels kind of naughty. In the winter, the newspapers are folded in the kindling box next to the wood stove.

As you would expect, spiritual subjects are popular at the ashram, and the library in the farmhouse caters to this taste. Swami Sivananda, who managed to write more than three hundred books, is well represented there, but not by all three hundred titles. Don't worry—there are enough of his works to hold you for quite a while. Naturally, books on yoga and Hinduism abound, but there are also books on all the major religions. Literature and poetry are there in abundance, as are encyclopedias. Though small, the library is packed from floor to ceiling with books. The filing system is haphazard. Unless you are looking for something by Swami Sivananda, the best approach is just to scan the shelves until something strikes your fancy. Looking for anything specific is guaranteed to give you a headache. I know, because I once spent an afternoon trying to organize the library. Reading is a popular pastime, though, and you are sure to see people spending their free hours, especially in cold weather, sitting near the fire absorbed in books. Reading about yoga is a good way to augment the practice, and every room has a copy of Swami Vishnu-Devananda's *Meditation and Mantras* on the bedside table. It is a most thorough and readable guide to meditating and an excellent choice for anyone who wants to make a lot of progress in one week. It's like the Gideon Bible of the ashram, except that you are not free to take it home. You can find it for sale in the boutique.

Shopping is not mentioned in the handbook, but browsing in the boutique is popular during its hours of operation. It is packed with books, yoga garb and mats, Sivananda T-shirts, sweatshirts, crystals, *mala* beads, incense, postcards, CDs and tapes, meditation shawls, and statues of deities. Allowances are made for junk-food junkies with a reasonable assortment of cookies, candy, potato chips, natural sodas, and ice cream made of rice milk. The boutique is like a halfway house for people suffering withdrawal symptoms from lack of shopping. There are no desserts at meals, unless someone has a birthday or it is a holiday, so those who are looking for some sugar can find it at the boutique. On weekends the boutique is a hangout for dedicated shoppers who need a quick fix.

All Roads Lead to the Sauna

Workshops and special programs are a mainstay at the ashram, and they are usually held in the temple on Saturdays and Sundays in the early afternoon. Usually they start around one o'clock, and they are often taught by visiting musicians, artists, diet experts, therapists of varying stripes, and religious leaders from wide-ranging traditions. Every weekend has a theme, and the workshops often run in tandem with the theme. For example, if Peruvian master flutist Jorge Alfano is giving a concert in sacred sounds at evening *satsang,* he will often give a Saturday afternoon workshop on traditional Andean music and instruments. Then on Sunday morning he will play those instruments at an Inca spiritual wheel ceremony at sunrise, held in place of the traditional morning *satsang.* Music workshops are frequent at the Ranch because Nada Yoga, the path of mystical union through sound, is such a powerful force, one that crosses all barriers of language and religious doctrines. Music can leap across cultural boundaries and allows us to enter new zones of spirit. The music workshops lean toward traditions in which music is a religious experience. A couple of workshop titles will give the idea: "Sacred Sounds: The Healing Process from Sound to Prayer" and "Inner Rhythms: Ancient Medicine for Modern Times." This is not even the tip of the iceberg when it comes to musical programs. The calendar is loaded with concerts and workshops. Devotional chanting, drumming, Nada Yoga, classical Indian dance, guitar, folk songs, and flute are just a few of the offerings.

Diet and health-oriented workshops come in a close second on the schedule, are held frequently, and are led by healers, herbalists, Ayurvedic practitioners, chiropractors, medical doctors, and others. Some of the titles give a fair idea of what is being offered: "Inner Transformation through Hatha Yoga," "Weekend Fast and Spring Cleaning," "Ayurveda

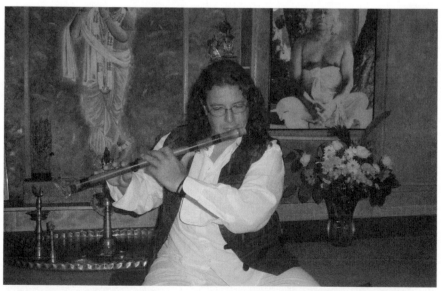

Music plays an important role in the yoga ashram. Here, master musician Jorge Alfano plays "sacred sounds" on a wide range of instruments from different traditions to demonstrate that in the diversity of cultures there is a unity of purpose.

for Self Care," "Learning to Detox," "Mind and Body Approach to Heal-ing," "*Asanas* as Yoga Therapy," "Stress Reduction," "Chiropractic Eval-uations and Exercises," "Massage for Yoga Practitioners," and so on. Holidays from all major religious traditions are celebrated with feasts and visiting spiritual leaders.

If you are staying for a week, the first couple of days you may find yourself being drawn back to your room for a nap. In the handbook's list of things to do in your free time, naps are in the "etcetera" catego-ry. Naps are wildly popular until people have become accustomed to the schedule. After a couple of days, the urge to sleep during the day begins to fade. Napping is not really considered a yogic activity. Sleep-ing during the day is considered to be *tamasic*. But in this high-pressure world it is very hard to get the kind of deep rest that is possible in the ashram. City dwellers are especially affected by the vegetarian diet and by all the fresh air they pump into and out of their lungs during *pranaya-ma*, the two-hour *asana* classes, and the meditation and chanting. As their minds begin to calm down, their eyelids get heavy. A commonly heard expression is "I just took the greatest nap." Some of the finest naps I have ever taken have been at the ashram. Free time is what it says it is, and if you want a nap you probably need it. If you are staying a week, there will be plenty of time for recreational napping.

If you want a truly world-class nap, I recommend that you take a sauna. I always take as many saunas as possible because the one at the Yoga Ranch is the real thing, and it feels so good. It's not one of these electric-powered redwood kits the size of a walk-in closet with design-er rocks on top. This is an authentic wood-fired sauna in the Russian style, full of character. Snugly dug into the side of a hill for insulation, it is spacious, comfortable, and rustic, with its own dressing room. There is nothing fancy about it, but it can easily bring a dozen or more people to a boil. When your muscles are sore from doing more Hatha Yoga than you are used to, that heat melts away any tension. There is even a window with a mountain view that stretches for miles. As you sweat out the toxins of modern life, you look out over the cool blueness of the mountains in the distance, and somehow you feel cooler. Nudity is not allowed, so bring a bathing suit. There is a cold shower in the corner, where you can bathe as long as you use biodegradable soap.

Standing beside the sauna is a woodshed the size of a one-car garage, filled with split oak to feed the sauna fire. The hungry firebox topped with boulders commands about a fourth of the interior of the sauna. A temperature gauge that looks as if it had come off a steam locomotive tells you exactly how hot you are. The hottest I ever saw it was 205 degrees, which is more than enough. Anything over 170 degrees is sufficient. When I am so hot that I can't take it any more, I go stand outside and let the steam vaporize off my lobster-red skin. Sometimes I jump in the pond just down the hill—unless it is covered with ice. Like the view, it takes your breath away. All that heat opens people up, and the conversations can be interesting. At the very least, they help you pass the time and bear the heat. Once I even got stock market tips from a Native American Indian shaman who said they had come to him in a dream. I didn't buy anything he recommended, but I followed them in the paper just to check it out. If I had bought the stock I would have made money. I have heard more than a few life stories in the sauna. When you are alone with another person, serious topics arise. When there are lots of people in there, it's like a general forum. Conversations start with the temperature of the sauna—that's like talking about the weather—and go on from there. The sauna is a place for bonding. You make friends in there as the heat strips off the body armor. People feel like coming clean—you can feel them lightening their loads.

A month after the disaster of September 11, I came to the Ranch to get away from the city. I live in downtown Manhattan, and the deadly odor emanating from the site and the deadening media coverage were getting to me. I could not stop watching the news. There is no television at the ashram except for videotapes. On my second day, I went into the sauna and saw a young man with a haggard and haunted face. I didn't ask him any questions, but I knew that he had been through a dreadful experience. We started to talk, and he said he was a New York City fireman trying to come to terms with the grief of losing fellow fire-fighters from his unit in Brooklyn, who had been some of the earliest on the scene. Before the first tower came down he was moving equipment near the foot of the building as dozens of jumpers hit the pavement around him. He said he was lucky they didn't land on him. When the building came down he had to run for his life. Every day for a month he had gone to the scene. At first he was looking for survivors; later he was searching for the remains of his fallen brothers. He was shaken up and had come to the ashram to heal his soul and his body, which had been poisoned by the fumes. "I don't know what else to do," he said. "I just walk around and talk to God."

As intimate as the sauna is, the major meeting place at the Ranch is the wide hall that separates the farmhouse from the temple. It functions like the lobby of a hotel. Of all the free time activities, hanging out in the hall, drinking herbal teas and talking, is probably the most popular. Sofas and chairs line the walls near the wood stove. You will be surprised how much you can learn about ashram life by just sitting there. It's like the corner of 42nd Street and Broadway. If you stay long enough, you will see everybody there. Conversation is easy, and anyone can join in—there's nothing snobby or cliquish about the place. You find yourself deeply engrossed with people you might never meet anywhere else. There is surprisingly little gossip, considering the close quarters, probably because sexuality is played down.

6

From Mind Control to Meditation

There having made the mind one-pointed, with the
actions of the mind and the senses controlled, let him,
seated on the seat, practice Yoga for the purification of
the Self.

—BHAGAVAD GITA

Yoga is restraining the activities of the mind.

—PATANJALI

When I first sit down in the morning to meditate in the temple at the
Yoga Ranch, I often try to revisit the dream I have just left behind. It
feels so close that I can smell it, but I want to see it again. I try to relo-
cate the dream area, but it swims away like a fish when poked at. I play
little games to retrieve the thread. I roll my eyes up and scan my mind
for dream-flavored images. (Why I roll the eyes I do not know, but it
seems to help.) Sometimes the dream does come back, but the recov-
ered dream feels manipulated and tamed. At first I am so involved in
this nostalgia for sleeping that I do not realize I am doing it. Then an

awareness of it dawns, and I observe my mind at work. This observation of the mind is not meditation itself, but it is a step in the right direction.

This is only one of the games my mind likes to play in the morning. Everything gathered in the mind during the night is there for inspection. Sitting cross-legged in the dark, I try to piece together images of memory still floating around from the movie I was dreaming when the bell rang. I observe this effort and tendency. I do not know whether this is a good thing to do or a distraction. It is said that truth is sometimes revealed in dreams and deep sleep and that progress in meditation can be made if one concentrates on the knowledge gained while dreaming. Sometimes I feel this is true. A black-and-white image appears, and I chase it like a dog bounding after a squirrel, and like a dog I give up slowly when the dream is up a tree and out of sight. Now I feel like a dog chasing its tail. I try to pull my attention away from the dream by shifting my inner focus to the place between my eyebrows. That is an inexact location. In the black field of my inner vision, this area occasionally has seemed to be a congregation point for light. I do not know what it is that I am supposed to see there. It's vague, as it is when I am teaching a yoga class and I tell the students, "Breathe into any areas of tension. Send your breath there." I know that it works, but I don't know how it works. I try to concentrate, but my mind wanders. I have to keep pulling it back. Then I begin to repeat the mantra and listen to it.

Concentration is enhanced when the mantra is used to time the breathing. For example, as you inhale you repeat mentally the words *Om Namah Sivaya* and then exhale those words. Then keep on doing that for thirty minutes, and see what happens. The mantra eats up other sounds. You fall into a zone where time is altered. Sometimes the half hour seems much shorter; sometimes it seems like eternity. The relationship of the mind and body is changed. They don't seem quite as separate. At the ashram, where meditation is done at the same time and place twice a day, progress is much more rapid. After a few days of uninterrupted *sadhana*, I find that I ride the mantra into meditation with full confidence that it will work.

Falling into Meditation

Swami Vishnu-Devananda in his book *Meditation and Mantras* uses the example of sleep to describe how to meditate. He says, "One may have a king-sized Posturepedic mattress, an air-conditioned room, and the absence of all disturbances, but sleep may not come. Sleep itself is not in anyone's hands. One falls into it. In the same way, meditation comes by itself. To still the mind and enter into the silence requires daily practice. Yet, there are certain steps that can be taken to establish a foundation and ensure success."

Swami Vishnu treated meditation in practical terms. His first rule for meditation was to set aside a regular place and time. At the ashram, nothing could be easier, but at home this is something that I need help with. At home, meditation competes with the urge to drink coffee and read a newspaper when I first wake up. Then an impulse might drive me toward the television just to get a peek at whatever appalling events might have occurred overnight. If something terrible has happened, I tend to leave the television news on. This is a *samskara* from my days as a newspaperman. When Jesus said, "Sufficient unto the day is the evil thereof," he was talking about not worrying about what is going to happen tomorrow. He meant that enough bad things are scheduled for today to keep you busy. The ashram is a refuge from distractions, a place where we can develop new and positive habits to replace the old ones. A *samskara* does not give ground to a vacuum. I once asked Swami Sitaramananda, who had been Swami Vishnu's personal secretary and is now the director of the Yoga Farm Ashram in northern

California, how to get rid of my bad habits. She is a tough-minded Viet-namese-born woman who was a girl during the war. Her answer was plain and straight: "You don't get rid of a bad habit. You make a good one to take its place." I consider this one of the most valuable bits of advice that anyone ever gave me. It came straight from the teachings of Swami Sivananda. He said, "You sow an action and reap a habit. You sow a habit and you reap a character. You sow a character and reap a destiny."

A week in an ashram gives us a break from our habits and lets us see them more clearly. This shift in perception is one of the greatest gifts that you can take home from a week of serious practice. I have never forgotten the way Henry Miller bemoaned in *The Tropic of Cancer* how he could never get all the dirt out of his navel. This image of meta-physical uncleanness stayed in my mind because I could identify with his frustration, but that is what an ashram does. It burns the dirt out of your navel. Washing alone will not do the job. This kind of dirt is really karma. It must be burnt, and the fire that burns it out is stoked by the practice of yoga.

The instant discipline supplied by the schedule and by a support group of others who share your ideals make it much easier to change old ways. The ashram does not provide instant enlightenment, but it removes the barriers and habits that separate you from your inner self. The atmosphere of safety provided by the ashram gives you the slack that allows you to unwind. Our lives can be like a tangled fishing line that can be untangled only by loosening the knots, not by pulling them tighter. The effects of this sense of security and purpose can be felt as the body armor of tension melts a little bit at a time. At home, I rebel against my dictates. At the ashram, all I have to worry about is getting out of bed. Once I am up, I am on my way. Getting up early is easier at the ashram, where human alarm clocks outside the room are bang-ing a gong at 5:30.

Opening the Inner Eye

All this talk about habits comes under the heading of mind control—really the first step toward successful meditation. The absence of an exciting night life is a big advantage on the spiritual path. If you go to bed at ten, getting up before dawn is a lot easier. The best time to meditate is called *Brahmamuhurta*, the hours between four and six in the morning. At this time of day, which many people never see, there is said to be a harmonious balance between the forces of light and darkness, day and night. The mind is fresh and unaffected by "the evil thereof." When the bell rings so early, worries have had less time to take hold, so concentration is easier to find. Sitting in the dim light, you feel closer to your true nature. At first, getting up early to meditate is a shock to the system; this is the old *samskaras* at work. A week at the ashram gives you the time to make some new *samskaras*. Positive habits can take root, but they may feel strange at first.

While the most important ingredient in successful meditation is a regular time, the place is very important. This time set aside for watching your mind at work is like watching a favorite TV show with no commercials. You make a regular date with yourself: same time, same place, your favorite chair. Pretty soon you have created a positive habit. If a special time and place are set aside, the mind finds it easier to be calm. Vibrations of peacefulness will gather in your special place. If you want, you can make yourself an altar with candles, incense, and the image of your chosen deity or inspirational figure. The best possible situation is to set aside a room to be used only for meditation and keep it locked. If space is tight, as it is in a typical New York City apartment, you can screen off an area. The main thing is to create a spiritual vibe and hold it. It sounds like a luxury, but this can be your place of refuge. Swami Vishnu-Devananda says that within six months your place of meditation will have a noticeable spiritual aura.

Such is the purpose of a temple. The temple is the heart of the ashram. The day begins and ends there. During the walk to the temple I feel the day begin. At the Ranch there is a short, delicious walk down the hill from the dormitory to the temple. I always scan the horizon on the way down. Off to the east a faint light appears at the horizon behind the distant ridge of mountains. I sniff the fresh *prana*-charged air. The morning energy is pure and unruffled. I feel rewarded just for being awake and happy in the knowledge of what is coming. Sometimes I can't wait to meditate. I want to bathe in the vibrations in the temple. This charge of sacred energy is the secret power of the ashram, the light that shines in the darkness and leads us to new beginnings. This transformation takes place during meditation. During meditation we close the deal between ourselves and God.

If you have never meditated before, the temple will help you begin auspiciously. If you are regular in your practice of meditation, you will feel the difference there. Simply being in a temple has the effect of jumpstarting the process of concentration. Practice with others is said to be more powerful than practice alone, especially in the early stages. There is also a feeling of safety in numbers. A subtle awareness dawns as you enter the temple and see others already sitting quietly. A spiritual practice needs to be nurtured in stillness at the beginning to take root. In unity we create a positive field of energy. You could say divinity loves company. This cumulative effect of so many serious aspirants practicing sincerely creates a zone of energy, and this spiritual momentum carries you along with it. You contribute to this sacred silence by not disturbing it, and you take something away from it by making noise. The peace in meditation is found in stillness. Eventually it all works out because people learn to be quiet when the noise someone else makes gets on *their* nerves. A little bit of self-control goes a long way. You notice this when the person behind you fidgets in nylon pants or takes the wrapper off a throat lozenge after a coughing spell.

Then there are the bottled water people, who make glugging sounds.

Temple etiquette boils down to respect. Swami Vishnu used to say that yoga begins when you take off your shoes. Before sitting, the correct thing to do is to prostrate by touching your forehead to the floor. This is a gesture of humility or reverence. When you do sit, find a comfortable cross-legged posture so that you will not have to keep moving around. You cannot hope to get anywhere in meditation if you can't sit still. At the very least, you will do your fellow aspirants a favor by curbing your impulses to squirm around and hawk your throat. People who ostentatiously try not to make noise can be very annoying. If you are late, just wait outside the temple until the chanting begins, and then enter. Sit down, relax, have a cup of tea, read a book, go back to sleep, whatever—but don't barge in after the meditation has started.

The reason for sitting in meditation with the legs crossed is not so that your hips and knees will feel pain, but because it makes a firm base for the body and creates a triangular path for the energy, *prana*, to travel so that it can gather at the base of the spine and not be dispersed in all directions. If you are not used to this way of sitting, your knees and hips may start to hurt before the half hour of meditation is over, and you will feel the need to move. You will not be the only one, and it is not a crime to move; just try to make as little noise as possible.

Here are a few more points to remember for keeping the space sacred. Sitting with the feet stretched out in front of you with the soles of your feet facing the altar is considered disrespectful, even though it is very natural to want to do it when your legs hurt. In many cultures, it is not polite to point the soles of your feet at other people. The same is true of the altar. One more foot *faux pas* is putting your foot on the prayer book. The more considerate you are, the more confident you will feel, in the same way that having good table manners will enhance your enjoyment of a banquet: instead of worrying about which fork to use, you can concentrate on more important things like the company. Finally, *prasad*, the food offering that ends every *satsang,* should be taken with the right hand and not the left.

On weekends at the ashram, simple instructions in how to meditate are given at the beginning of *satsang,* because that is when most first-
time visitors come. Swami Padmapananda enters, bows to the altar, and
sits. At exactly six o'clock he repeats "Om" three times, and everyone
joins in. "Sit up straight in a comfortable cross-legged position with your
back at a ninety-degree angle to the floor," he says. His voice is steady
and calm. He has given these instructions thousands of times, but he
has not tired of giving them. "Close your eyes and bring your concentration to the point between your eyebrows if you are primarily an intellectual, or thinking, person. If you are mostly devotional, or loving, bring
your attention to the place at the center of the heart. Both places are
equally good; so choose the one that seems best for you, and once
you have chosen your place of concentration, the one that you think
is best, stay with it."

The reason for not changing your point of focus is explained by a
metaphor from Swami Sivananda. If you want to reach water when digging a well, you are more likely to succeed by digging one deep well
than by digging many shallow ones. By now I have heard these instructions many times, but each time I hear them I do what he says. I'm
not sure that I am an intellectual, but it's a closer description than devotional, so I keep picking the place between my eyebrows. The *ajna chakra*
is located there, and meditating there is said to destroy the karma of past
lives and bestow intuition. The *chakra* in the heart area is called the *ana-
hata,* and meditation there is said to bestow cosmic love and psychic
powers. I adjust my posture so that my back will be straight as the swami
continues.

"Once you have chosen a point, shift your awareness to your breathing. Make the inhalation and exhalation equal in length. Try to make
your breathing as soft and subtle as possible. Inhale . . . one . . . two . . .
three, and exhale . . . one . . . two . . . three. If you have a personal mantra,

repeat it silently to yourself to regulate the breathing. If you do not have a personal mantra, you can use the universal mantra: Om. Try to let go of any thoughts of yesterday or worries about tomorrow. If thoughts come into your mind, just observe them and let them pass. If your mind starts to wander, gently bring the attention back to your breathing, and focus on the point of concentration that you have chosen. Now adjust your posture and try to do this for the next half an hour."

Then his voice stops, and there is silence. When I meditate, my mind wanders a good deal of the time, and I am sure that this is true of anyone who has tried to meditate. Sometimes I wonder if there is something wrong with the way my mind works, because it is so hard to control. Some of the things that come into my mind are trivial or embarrassing, and others are shameful. Whatever comes up is there to be observed.

"Through meditation, play of the mind is witnessed," says Swami Vishnu-Devananda. "In the early stages, nothing can be done other than to gain understanding as the ego is observed constantly asserting itself. But in time its games become familiar, and one begins to prefer the peace of contentment."

Controlling the Mind-Stuff

Swami Vishnu taught students preparing for meditation to command the mind to remain quiet for a specified amount of time. Unruly as the mind can be, it will relax and comply with discipline for a reasonable length of time. If you were to say to the mind, "Be quiet forever!" the mind would ignore the request, but if you say, "Be quiet for half an hour," it will take the bait. This sounds funny, but it is worth trying. There is nothing crazy about talking to yourself in this way. The subconscious mind will respond to direct requests of this sort. You can prove this by telling yourself to wake up at a certain time. Tell yourself to get up at

six, and you will do it—maybe not the first time, but if you keep working with your subconscious, it will work with you. This consciousness
that you are talking to is called *chitta* in Sanskrit. *Chitta* can be compared
to the hard drive of our cosmic computer. Everything is on it. Sometimes
it is translated as "mind-stuff." According to yogic teachings, this *chitta*
stays with us forever—not only from birth to death, but from life to
life. It is the source of feelings, memories (from this life and all previous
lives), and the ego. *Chitta* also includes the spiritual heart and is said to
be located there—not in the physical heart but to the right of the physical heart in the astral body. In his *Ayurveda and the Mind*, Dr. David Frawley outlines the broad territory of this subtle substance. "*Chitta* is the
most intimate and enduring part of our being. It is the mind of the soul,
the individualized portion of the Divinity that we are."

Chitta is the object of the sage Patanjali's famous definition of yoga,
"*Yogas chitta-vritti nirodhah*," which is translated as "Yoga is restraining the activities of the mind." This deceptively simple sentence is the
first premise of Raja Yoga and a common denominator for what takes
place at any Sivananda ashram. It is the dividing line between what is
to be done and what is not to be done. That which lends to restraining the activities of the mind is encouraged, and that which tends to
inflame the mind is discouraged. Patanjali compiled his sayings on
how to control the mind in the second century B.C.E. These ideas were
already established in the Vedas, but his interpretation refreshed them,
and their relevance has not been diminished by time. Patanjali's *Yoga-
Sutras* were written at a time when most people could not read and
write. He wrote in a style that could be memorized and passed down
by word of mouth. The instructions for controlling the mind are almost
a training manual.

Patanjali's *Yoga-Sutras* survive today in numerous translations and
commentaries because they appeal to the skeptical, modern mind. In
his *Raja Yoga*, Swami Vivekananda, a disciple of Ramakrishna and a great

skeptic himself, says, "So far then, we see that in the study of Raja Yoga no faith or belief is necessary. Believe nothing until you find it out for yourself; that is what it teaches us. Truth requires no prop to make it stand." These comments were made in a lecture given in the 1920s in New York and were put into book form. Since then, Vivekananda's *Raja Yoga* has been reprinted twenty-six times, most recently in the year 2000. I have four translations of *Yoga–Sutras* in my library. In addition to Vivekananda's version, Swami Vishnu-Devananda includes a version in his *Meditation and Mantras*. I like them both for different reasons. Perhaps my new favorite is *How to Know God: The Yoga Aphorisms of Patanjali* by Swami Prabhavananda and Christopher Isherwood, published in 1952. I find it easier to assimilate because Isherwood, who wrote the excellent *Ramakrishna and His Disciples*, is English and bridges the culture gap. Finally, there is a version by T. K. V. Desikachar that was first published in 1987 and is nice and short—just over one hundred pages with commentary. So you can see that there is an enduring interest in this ancient classic.

The yoga practiced at any Sivananda ashram today would be familiar to Patanjali. Swami Vishnu-Devananda's endorsement is unequivocal: "Raja Yoga, the royal path of mind control, is the most comprehensive and scientific approach to God-Realization. The precepts and doctrines of this ancient science were first compiled and explained by Patanjali Maharishi, the greatest psychologist of all time. Never has man's mind been so completely analyzed. Never has a process for eliminating human woes and frailties been so succinctly presented. The methods of Raja Yoga are profoundly timeless. Though of ancient origin, they are still the most useful technique available to modern man beset by tremendous stresses and strains of competitive society."

What I find so engaging and satisfying about the *Yoga-Sutras* is how Patanjali lays out such a practical course. Belief is not necessary, but practice is. He describes the process of reaching the state of superconscious

God-realization step by step, almost like building a house. After the time I've spent reading different *Yoga-Sutras* translations and commentaries, it has slowly dawned on me that to Patanjali, self-realization is no pie-in-the-sky dream. *Samadhi* is real to Patanjali. Knowing that at the ashram, the yoga taught springs from such an ancient source reassures me that these practices are the real thing, especially when they still generate so much interest. For a system to last for thousands of years, it must reflect some enduring truth. The idea is not simply "Gimme that old-time religion; it's good enough for me."

The First Steps of Raja Yoga

Yoga has a way of reinventing itself without losing its true nature. The way yoga adapts to changing times could almost be called sly. Yoga is spirituality flying under the radar. When people who are very body-conscious discover yoga, they often get more than they bargained for. They start off with a physical pursuit and end up with a lot more. A good example of how this works can be seen in the evolution of the San-skrit word *Astanga*. For a couple of thousand years, *Astanga*, which in Sanskrit means "eight-limbed," was another name for Patanjali's system of Raja Yoga because it is divided into eight parts. When people say *Astanga* now, they are probably talking about a strenuous type of Hatha Yoga developed by the south Indian Hatha Yoga master Pattabhi Jois. Western students flock to his Ashtanga Research Institute in Mysore to study with this eighty-plus master on the concrete floor of his home. Instead of holding steady postures, students do a continuous series of movements that are synchronized with the breath, something like the Sun Salutation but more difficult and elaborate. According to Jois's system, as the student progresses the physical and astral bodies become purer, the *prana* builds, and eventually the *kundalini* is awakened and *samadhi* is achieved. The goal is the same, but the means are different.

Sitting meditation is not what this yoga is about. Jois says, "Sit still and you get monkeys in the head." One need not go to India to find this system of *Astanga*. It is taught everywhere now.

Restraint is considered to be the most basic power for a yogi to possess. Power over one's self is the first step. Patanjali listed five restraints, or *yamas*, as the first of *Astanga*'s eight limbs. The *yamas* are much like the Commandments of the Hebrew scripture. The first of these restraints is *ahimsa:* to do no harm to any living creature by thought, word, or deed. This corresponds to "Thou shalt not kill." The knowledge that we cannot hurt others without hurting ourselves is the force that gives life to the Golden Rule: "Do unto others as you would have them do unto you." Because *ahimsa* applies to all living things and not just humans, yogic diet is vegetarian for ethical as well as health reasons. Swami Vivekananda said, "The test of *ahimsa* is the absence of jealousy." Such a view of noninjury is a long way from merely not killing. Envy and jealousy are the enemies of concentration.

The second restraint is to always tell the truth: *satya.* Jesus said, "The truth shall set you free." Honesty is the best policy because it is the most liberating. Lying is such a burden that truthfulness becomes a necessity. It is impossible to get anywhere on the spiritual path if you are a liar, because you are also lying to yourself. The need for truthfulness is easy to understand. At times we have all woven tangled webs and destroyed our peace of mind. We have all been burned by not telling the truth. To say that it messes up our meditation would be the least of our problems.

The third *yama*, sexual restraint, is called *brahmacharya.* It opposes the modern view that the body is personal property as long as no one else is hurt. *Brahmacharya* is concerned with wider issues as well: with energy as well as ethics. Sexual yearnings do not coexist easily with a calm mind. *Brahmacharya* asserts that a higher level of consciousness is possible when sexual energy is sublimated. The *Yoga-Sutras* say, "When a man becomes steadfast in his abstention from incontinence, he acquires spiritual energy."

Perhaps it would be best to let a swami speak on the benefits of sexual restraint. "Now we come to a very sticky one, *brahmacharya*," says Swami Padma. He is giving a workshop on the obstacles to meditation in the temple at the Yoga Ranch. "I could talk about this all day. *Brahmacharya* means controlling all the senses, but the hardest one to control is the sexual instinct, because it is an instinct. It depends on your vision, or aspiration in life. How far do you want to go on the spiritual path? It's not easy—the odds are against you in the modern world. Look at advertising. It is designed to make you more passionate. It gets worse and worse. I'm not trying to be a prude. What you do is your own business. It only matters if your aspirations are high. I was not born a *brahmachari*—quite the opposite—but as I practice I see that it works. It depends on what level of joy you want to experience in your *sadhana.* If you want to get to a higher level, you have to make some sacrifices. Sometimes when I am flooded with grace I look to God with thanks. I want more and more of that. To get that grace I am willing to make those sacrifices. You need to be aware of the tremendous power of our sexual nature and use some discrimination. It can turn your life upside down. If you have some sexual feelings, prostrate yourself to that person mentally, and if that doesn't work try it again with more feeling. You control your senses like you become a vegetarian, bit by bit. You start in small ways by being more moderate, by thinking about the advantages of having a pure mind and not having this bother you all the time. When I wake up I thank God that I am still on this path."

The fourth *yama*, not stealing, is called *asteya*. It also includes not coveting and not being jealous. While the advantages of nonstealing are apparent to most of us, Patanjali says there is a reward. "When a man becomes steadfast in his abstention from theft," he says, "all wealth comes to him." About this, Vivekananda made a wry comment: "The more you fly from nature, the more she follows you, and if you do not care for her at all, she becomes your slave." The fifth and final *yama* is not taking bribes or accepting gifts. Patanjali says that if a man is completely free of greed he will be able to remember all his past, present, and future lives.

A swami is asked, "What do you think about reading the thoughts of others?" He answers, "I think it is impolite." Powers like this are called *siddhi*s. These powers have a strong allure, and they are easy to abuse. They are regarded as tests of will and serve as signals to the aspirant that he or she is on the right path. If you start reading peoples' minds and seeing the future, you would do well to keep these powers to yourself and not use them to impress others, because they can be a trap. What fascinates me about these powers is that their source is said to be in the practice of the *yama*s.

There are seven more limbs to *Astanga*. The *yama*s are the first rung on the spiritual ladder. The second rung consists of spiritual practices, the *niyama*s, and there are five of them. These are spiritual practices. The *niyama*s are about the observances of worship. Whereas the *yama*s are about ethics, the *niyama*s are about purification and expressions of devotion. The first of the *niyama*s is *saucha,* or purity. Washing yourself when you get up in the morning is *saucha,* and purity of thought is just as important. Next comes contentment, or *santosha*. Without contentment our mind is forever restless. If yoga is the practice of controlling the mind, it is clearly impossible without contentment. Our contentment is under constant attack by those who would sell us something. We are brainwashed by advertising into thinking that contentment can be bought. Yoga says that contentment is the nature of the eternal Self. The third concept, *tapas,* or austerity, is familiar. It is expressed by fasting. The logic of *tapas* is that by denying comfort to the body, one fans the flames of spirit. Swami Vishnu-Devananda, however, warned that too much concern with denying the body was a sign that a person was too concerned about the body in general. We are in danger of pride when we make sacrifices. The fourth *niyama*, studying religious books, is called *swadhyaya*. A certain amount of time each day should be spent elevating the mind with religious texts. Reading religious books prepares the devotee for *Ishwara-pranidhana*, the fifth *niyama:* surrendering the ego to God. All the *yamas* and *niyamas* come down to this. All the restraints and observances make it possible. It is said that Raja Yoga begins where the ego ends.

All the Way to Samadhi

The third step on the ladder of Raja Yoga is the part of yoga that everyone knows about: the practice of *asanas*. In Raja Yoga, the *asanas* are a means to an end, and not an end in themselves. They are the vehicle that carries the aspirant to higher levels. Patanjali does not say much about the practice of *asanas*, but what he does say is simple and direct: "*Asanas* should be steady and comfortable." Swami Vishnu-Devananda, a master of Hatha Yoga, explains the meaning like this: "Hatha Yoga postures, always done in a specific order, massage the endocrine glands and release energy blockages in the body so that a meditative state is brought about physically rather than sitting and watching the mind." The emphasis is on steadiness and comfort, because these will allow the body to relax and free the mind for concentration. Patanjali rounds out his discussion of *asanas* by saying, "Posture is mastered by releasing tension and meditating on the Unlimited." By practicing *asanas* from a spiritual perspective, the yogi is able to master the postures and opens up in ways that transcend limitations.

Pranayama is the fourth limb of *Astanga*. The literal meaning of *pranayama* is restraint of *prana*. Controlling *prana* is like controlling the life force. The great Hatha yogi B. K. S. Iyengar in his *Light on Pranayama* says, "It is as difficult to explain *prana* as it is to explain God." *Prana* has many aspects; among them are breath, energy, strength, and life. *Ayama* means restraint, or control. In practice, *pranayama* means restraint or control of the breath and life force. The two *pranayamas* performed are *kapalabathi* (shining skull) and *analoma viloma* (alternate-nostril breathing). Both can be practiced without fear, but the more advanced forms should be undertaken with a teacher who understands the subject deeply. They can dangerous unless the body and mind are pure. I have heard stories of students who went off the deep end after practicing advanced *pranayamas* without proper instruction. Iyengar says, "The practice of *pranayama* develops a steady mind, strong willpower, and sound judgment."

It is said that the mind has two impulses. One is to merge with the senses by directing the attention outward, and the other is to look inward and merge with the self. The withdrawal of the senses from sensual attractions is called *pratyahara,* and it is the fifth limb of *Astanga.* Patanjali says, "*Pratyahara* is the imitation of the mind by the senses, which comes from withdrawing the senses from their objects." We are under such a heavy bombardment of sensual stimulation that it is easy to see why it would be helpful to be able to pull back from it. Our desires are not extinguished by gratification. Yoga's answer to this wheel of misfortune is to train the mind to disengage from the senses and change the focus inward.

The final three limbs of Raja Yoga are *dharana, dhyana,* and *samadhi.* Taken together, they are the three highest levels of meditation, called *samyama.* The first of them, *dharana,* is fixing the mind on one object. It is said that if the mind can maintain a constant unbroken flow of attention to an object for twelve seconds, this is *dharana,* or concentration. Vivekananda gives these instructions for concentration: "The mind should think of one point in the heart. That is very difficult; an easier way is to imagine a lotus there. That lotus is full of light. Effulgent light. Put the mind there."

The next level is meditation, or *dhyana*. *Dhyana* and *dharana* are both concentration; the difference is in how long they can be held. In *dhyana*, the concentration is unbroken for twelve times twelve seconds: about two and a half minutes.

The highest level of meditation is called *samadhi*, or absorption. *Samadhi* is said to be a continuous flow of attention for twelve times twelve times twelve seconds, or about half an hour, but there is much more to it than that. There is a difference in the quality of the meditation. Here the observer is merged into the object of attention, and the only awareness is that they are one. This is a state of oceanic bliss of unity with the universe, and from the yogic perspective there is no higher state of existence. Now it might seem that we have come to the end of the line, but this is not the case. The great sage Brahmananda declared, "Spiritual life begins after *samadhi*."

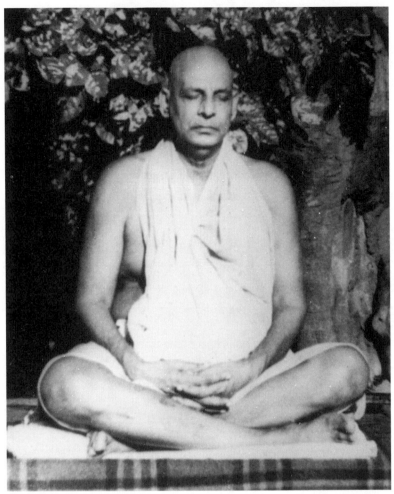

Swami Sivananda, the great turn-of-the-century Indian saint, founded a yoga empire based on selfless service. After a highly successful career as a doctor running a hospital for the families of poor miners in Malaya, Swami Sivananda renounced the world and founded an ashram in the Himalayas. His disciple, Swami Vishnu-Devananda, carried the torch of Karma Yoga to the West and founded many ashrams.

7

Work Is Worship

*Do thou always without attachment perform action
which should be done; for by performing action without
attachment, man reaches the Supreme.*

—BHAGAVAD GITA

The title of this chapter is a saying of Swami Sivananda, and the
Bhagavad Gita verse quotes Krishna. Work is worship. That says it all.
The first time I heard the writings of Swami Sivananda was at *satsang*.
His *Bliss Divine* was often read after the chanting. The book is a series
of inspiring essays alphabetically arranged from A to Z. As inspirational
reading, *Bliss Divine* lives up to its name. Open it at random and it pours
out wisdom, often on a topic that relates to an issue that is on your
mind. For instance, the letter A is represented by *ahimsa*: "*Ahimsa* is not
mere negative noninjuring. It is positive cosmic love." The letter K has
a tightly edited, nine-page entry on karma. "Any physical or mental
action is karma. Thinking is mental karma. Karma is the sum total of
our acts, both in the present life and in the preceding births."

I did not have to be an editor for more than twenty years to appreciate how much Swami Sivananda could say with a few words. He had
a bold way with words that traveled well from East to West. Born in
1887 to a pious Brahmin family and educated as a doctor, he was well

equipped for spreading the gospel of yoga. He never set foot in the United States, but two of his many disciples had major roles in bringing yoga to North America. Swami Vishnu-Devananda has already been mentioned. Swami Satchidananda, who founded Integral Yoga in the United States, was also initiated as a swami in Rishikesh by Swami Sivananda. Integral Yoga follows the same precepts as Sivananda. The name "Integral" underscores the ecumenical approach of welcoming all faiths as paths to the same light. The shared theme is "Unity in Diversity."

The organization founded by Swami Satchidananda has its headquarters in central Virginia on the James River. A spectacular lotus-shaped temple graces the ashram. Inside are altars representing all faiths. Yogaville is the name of this planned community and ashram situated on almost a thousand acres. Although I grew up in nearby Richmond, I recently visited for the first time and was surprised to find that the main building was Sivananda Hall, just as at the Ranch. I realized then that Swami Sivananda's influence was wider than I had imagined. Integral Yoga has a major center in Manhattan on West 13th Street, half a block from where I live. The center offers a full roster of classes and special programs. I have taken Hatha Yoga classes there and have found them traditional and effective. Integral Yoga also has an organic grocery store, where I shop all the time, and a well-stocked bookstore with a great vegetarian cookbook section. Swami Satchidananda is in his eighties now, and his organization is thriving as never before. Integral Yoga also has an ashram in Tamil Nadu, South India. Swami Sivananda planted seeds of good karma in his disciples, and now we are able to harvest it.

The Practice of Karma Yoga

All this success is the result of intense Karma Yoga. Service builds a shelter for other ideals. The basic unit of service is the individual, but the ashram is the ideal nurturing place for Karma Yoga. The language of service is understood the world over. The practitioners have followed Swami Sivananda's dictum: "Adapt. Adjust. Accommodate." Ashrams survive on that mandate.

I like books that you can pick up and start reading in the middle. A random passage from *Bliss Divine* has always managed to hit the mark. Sivananda's ability with words reminds me of H. L. Mencken's definition of journalism as "the art of turning clichés into finely honed epigrams." I was amazed that his words could embed themselves in my head without annoying me. That is the major test of a mantra. (Sometimes insipid songs from the radio also rattle around in there.) In three little words he lays the foundation for Karma Yoga: "Work is worship. Work is meditation. Serve all with intense love without any idea of agency and without expectation of fruits or reward." This way of looking at work makes sense. His understanding gives off light. The statement rings with truth because modern life is so much about work. Our egos are so tied up in the work we do. We define ourselves by what we do for a living.

Swami Sivananda was a medical doctor. His work took him out of the ivory tower and put him in contact with the world. His medical practice gave him the opportunity to serve in Malaya, where he ran a hospital for poor miners and their families. But the spiritual life was calling for his full attention, and at the height of his medical career he returned to India and became a wandering monk. In 1924 he was initiated into *sannyasa* at the age of thirty-seven. For years he practiced strict austerity in the solitude of the Himalayan jungles, but in 1936 he heard a calling and founded the Divine Life Society, dedicated to spreading spiritual knowledge. Somehow he also wrote more than three hundred books in his lifetime. Someone asked him what those books were all about. His answer was six words: "Serve. Love. Give. Purify. Meditate. Realize." He put service first and realization last because he knew that the process worked. "Karma Yoga prepares the mind for the reception of light, or knowledge," he said. "It expands the heart and breaks all barriers that stand in the way of unity or oneness."

Karma is a daunting subject, and I suspected I needed help writing about it. I vaguely recalled that Swami Sivananda had written a book about karma, but I didn't know the title. On a matter as weighty as karma I was certain there had to be something, and I was not disappointed. I scanned the shelves of the library at the Ranch and found exactly the book I was looking for: *The Practice of Karma Yoga*, in 204 pages. There was more in there about karma than I wanted to know, but as I read the book I began to understand it from the point of view of the tradition that defined the word.

Thanks to Karma Yoga, I came in contact with the literary Sivananda. Not all his books are found on the shelves of the Ranch's library, but there are plenty. One rainy day I organized them. That was an enlightening few hours, delightful too because the library was so cozy that afternoon. The two windows were streaked with rain. One of them had in it a lacy wood carving of Siva Nataraj, the dancing Shiva. The desk had a computer hooked up to the Internet, and all the walls were lined floor to ceiling with books. To be in a small, warm room surrounded by books on a drizzly winter day is to know something about contentment. The smell of dry books lined up on all sides between me and the damp world outside made me thankful. Srinivasan had suggested that it would be a good idea if all Swami Sivananda's books for sale in the boutique were also available in the library to be read for free. I listed every title in the library and found that dozens of books for sale in the boutique were unavailable from the library. Nevertheless, there were still scores of books on the shelves by Sivananda. That day gave me some insight into the breadth of Swami Sivananda's writing.

The depth of his work would take years to explore. He had taken on all the big topics. His voice sings with real spiritual authority. The books are actually inspiring. If you were to read all his works, you would have a complete education about yoga. Occasionally, the comparisons are dated. A woman was rarely a swami when the books were first published, and some references cast females in the category of temptresses, obstacles on the spiritual path rather than leaders. The lapses are of the time and not in his heart. Swami Sivananda's reach was great, but it did not exceed his grasp. He built bridges between the ancient East and the New World that still stand, spanning ignorance to connect bodies of thought. Much of his work is still in print and is published by the Divine Life Society he founded. An example of his vocal style is found in this warning that karma is no excuse for fatalism: "Do not say: 'Karma, karma. My karma has brought me like this.' Exert. Exert. Do Purusharta [self effort]. Do Tapas [practice austerity]. Concentrate. Purify. Meditate. Do not become a fatalist. Do not yield to inertia. Do not bleat like a lamb. Roar *Om, Om, Om* like a lion of Vedanta." I have a cassette tape on which he says these words in a powerful voice during a *satsang*. When you read them you may feel they are excessive, but spoken they are electrifying. Swami Sivananda left the body in 1963, which makes the tape at least forty years old. The rhythm of his speech is evangelistic. He roars like a lion of Vedanta.

Laying Down the Law

It is the fate of karma to give birth to many studies and to be a subject of great interest to *pandits*. The *pandits* are Sanskrit scholars who interpret the scriptures. The English word *pundit* (one who comments on current affairs) is derived from it. These days, pundits are the newspaper columnists and news people who yell over each other on talk shows, but they had a sacred beginning: explaining the meaning behind religious works. *Pandits* wrote and still do write commentaries on ancient texts such the *Bhagavad Gita* (Song of God), and many are holy people.

You would not call Swami Sivananda a *pandit* because he was a *jivan-mukta*, a Self-Realized saint. However, like a *pandit,* he wrote commentary on a wide range of religious texts and topics.

Much of what he has to say about Karma Yoga and karma comes from the *Bhagavad Gita,* in which the laws of Karma come to life in the advice given by Krishna to Arjuna on how to act on the battlefield—a battlefield not unlike daily existence. As I delved into Swami Sivananda's *Practice of Karma Yoga,* I saw that there is more to karma than I had ever imagined. I decided to let Swami Sivananda's writings be my guide through the intricate maze of karma and Karma Yoga. The path led me to the *Bhagavad Gita,* the mother lode on the subject of karma. The translation I had at home was by Swami Sivananda, with commentary so useful that it could be called essential for understanding this essential text.

The *Gita* is all about duty. Krishna tells Arjuna what he must do. "O Arjuna, work incessantly. Your duty is to work always. But do not expect fruits. The lot of man who expects fruits is pitiable indeed! He is the most miserable man in the world." In Karma Yoga, virtue is its own reward. The fruits of work are like the fragrance of flowers. On great occasions in India, baskets of flowers are thrown in handfuls to the altar or at the feet of the guru during worship. These ceremonies are called *pujas.* Before the annual *puja* honoring the *Mahasamadhi* day of Swami Vishnu-Devananda, the Teachers Training Course group was given instructions on how to show devotion. Our guide to the ceremony was Swami Govindananda, a Keralan from the south of India, where flowers are abundant and used with abandon at religious festivals. To prepare us for what would happen at the *puja,* he said, "Someone will come and fill your hands with flowers. You will want to do this." He lowered his head and sniffed loudly, then looked up and smiled. "But don't do it. The fragrance is not for you."

Karma Comes in All Sizes

Everyone thinks they know what karma is, and basically they are correct. The law of karma is fully imbedded in our collective unconscious. Karma gives us some of our most time-tested slogans: "You get what you give." "Do unto others as you would have them do unto you." "Everything that goes around comes around." "No good deed goes unpunished." "You reap what you sow." These are just a few. Like everyone else, I think I know something about karma. There is a school of hard knocks, and we all attend it at times, some more than others. This is where we learn Karma 101, the law of retribution. "He who robs another man, robs himself first. He who hurts another man, hurts himself first. He who cheats another man, cheats himself first," says Sivananda. The law of retribution teaches us lessons we will never forget.

The concept that divine justice will prevail and eventually even all scores is accepted in many religions, but the Hindus take the ball and run with it. There are as many kinds of karmas as there are yogas. According to Vedantic literature, there is so much karma that it takes thousands of lifetimes to work it all out, and it *will* be worked out. In Hindu thought, karma occupies a position similar to the central location of gravity in scientific thought. Both represent inexorable laws, and both give rise to a great deal of speculation. The word *karma* evolved from the Sanskrit root *kri,* meaning "action" or "deed." Anything that has consequences creates karma. The deed and the results of the deed are the same thing. Action and reaction are the same. Thoughts are also considered to be actions; in fact, thoughts are considered to have a reality surpassing that of solid objects. You can run, but you can't hide from them. People, it is said, see actions. God sees motives.

The doctrine of karma includes the law of action and reaction, the law of compensation, and the law of retribution. These laws are considered to be immutable and forever unchanging. The law of action and reaction is precise and almost mathematical in its inevitability. When it says that there is a reaction for every action, be sure that the reaction comes with equal force. This law oversees the fruits of previous actions. Karma is like a banking system. You only get out of it what you put into it. The law of compensation brings balance into nature. "If there are ten scoundrels in a place there are two sattvic souls to bring compensation," writes Sivananda, adding, "If there is a flood-tide at Puri, there is an ebb-tide at Waltair. This is the law of compensation. If there is day in India, there is night in America. Peace follows a war, and vice versa. This is the law of compensation." On the law of retribution he says, "There is nothing chaotic or capricious in this world. Things do not happen in this universe by accident or chance in a disorderly manner. They happen in regular succession. They follow each other in regular order. There is a certain definite connection between what is done now by you and what will happen in the future. Sow always the seeds which will make pleasant fruits and which will make you happy, herein and hereafter."

Karma can be divided into three kinds, *Sanchita, Prarabdha,* and *Agami.* The first, *Sanchita,* is all the accumulated karmas from the past, including all past lives. This is the karma that is expressed in a person's character and tendencies. The second kind of karma, *Prarabdha,* is past action that is ripe and ready to be reaped. This is the special karma that you have taken this particular body to experience. There is no way out of it. Even a *jivanmukta* is not immune to this kind of karma. He or she also must live in the human body. *Prarabdha* karma is payback time. *Agami* is the fresh karma you are making right this minute and storing away to be dealt with in the future.

Swami Sivananda uses a classic metaphor in *Bliss Divine* to characterize the three kinds of karma. "In Vedantic literature there is a beautiful analogy," he writes. "The bowman has already sent an arrow; it has left his hands. He cannot recall it. He is about to shoot another arrow. The bundle of arrows in the quiver on his back is the *Sanchita.* The arrow he has just shot is *Prarabdha*. And the arrow he is about to shoot from his bow is *Agami*. Of these he has perfect control over the *Sanchita* and *Agami*, but he must surely work out his *Prarabdha*. The past which has begun to take effect he has to experience."

The first three chapters of the *Bhagavad Gita* are devoted to karma. These chapters are dedicated to the necessity of doing your duty, even when the situation is confusing and ambiguous. The situation is fraught with danger in the first chapter. The great general Arjuna is hesitating on the field of battle. He is in despair because he has family, friends, and teachers on both sides. Dejectedly, he drops his bow and sits down, not knowing what to do. The good news for Arjuna is that Krishna is there with him. To clear up the confusion, Krishna gives Arjuna this instruction in the second chapter. "Thou hast grieved for those that should not be grieved for, yet thou speakest words of wisdom," says Krishna. "The wise grieve neither for the living, nor for the dead." Krishna's advice reminds Arjuna that the self is eternal and that the soul takes on new bodies. "These bodies of the embodied Self, which is eternal, indestructible, and immeasurable, are said to have an end. Therefore fight, O Arjuna." Krishna tells Arjuna that his duty is to fight, to act. "Thy right is to work only, but never with its fruits; let not the fruits of action be thy motive, nor let this attachment be to inaction." By focusing on the task at hand and not thinking about glory or defeat, Krishna lays out the means for Arjuna to understand how to do his duty. Krishna does not tell Arjuna to stand on his head and meditate. Karma Yoga is called skill in action. "Perform action, O Arjuna, being steadfast in yoga, abandoning attachment and balanced in success and failure. Evenness of mind is called yoga." The *Gita* says that motive is a major factor in whether or not one is doing the right thing. If you are concerned with gain and loss, you are not giving the fruits of your actions to God. The *Gita* leaves no doubt that when the time comes to act, it is wrong to do nothing. Krishna says to Arjuna, "Not by nonperformance of actions does a man reach actionlessness; nor by mere renunciation does he attain to perfection." How does this life-and-death situation of a great battle relate to the day-to-day chores at the ashram? It's a daily struggle, and Krishna brings it down to earth when he says, "Do thou perform [thy] bounden duty, for action is superior to inaction, and even the maintenance of the body would not be possible for thee by inaction."

Will Work for Yoga

The ashram is like a body, and it requires constant maintenance. The hands and feet of this body are unpaid Karma yogis. Without the self-less service of Karma yogis, the ashram could not survive. To live up to its utopian ideals, the ashram calls on staff members who trade their energy, time, and talents to live at the ashram full time. These full-time Karma yogis must sign up for at least a month of service, but many stay longer and some stay much longer. The ashram is nourished by a steady trickle of people who want to go full time with yoga and are willing to work five hours a day to cover their expenses. The Yoga Ranch always has a few transient staffers who round out a full-time contingent at the ashram. The number changes almost constantly as people come and go. People stay a while, leave, and come back. The Sivananda organization moves key people around where they can have the most impact, or where they might like to go. It's almost like an army of Karma yogis who spread information on yoga.

Despite its worldwide scope, there is a good deal of contact among the original disciples of Swami Vishnu-Devananda, who now run the organization by committee. On the ashram level, the microcosm, the staff is like a loose family, with Srinivasan and his wife, Laksmi, as leaders. They represent a benign authority and make the important decisions. Srinivasan, whose father was a schoolmaster, has the look of a college dean. Sri has been the director and Laksmi the codirector at the Ranch for eight years. Laksmi and Sri have an interesting dynamic balance. She is a frank, funny Frenchwoman and master teacher of Hatha Yoga. He is of a philosophical nature, so the karmic law of compensation has ordained that he must keep the light of Karma Yoga lit and keep peace among the staff.

Every morning after *satsang* there is a staff meeting to plan the day ahead. Guests do not attend this meeting. Duties are assigned with regard to fairness, but as Swami Sivananda said, "Every work is a mixture of good and evil. There can be neither absolute good work nor absolute bad work in this world. This physical universe is a relative place. If you do some action, it will do some good in one corner, and some evil in another corner. You must try to do such actions that can bring the maximum of good and the minimum of evil." If there is any deviation from the duty roster posted in the kitchen, this staff meeting is when it gets worked out. Sometimes the best-laid plans must change. Meanwhile, there are usually a few staff situations boiling to stir the pot.

Ashram life attracts a wide range of personalities who have to work together and get along with one another. Friction is inevitable at times. It starts as an undercurrent, something like this: Tejas is tired of working in the laundry and wants to take care of the altar. Shakti does not like to vacuum and make beds but loves to cook. Narayani says that Shakti puts too many chilies in the soup. Ganesha feels that he gets stuck with phone duty more than anyone else. He wants to feed the cows for a change. Gauri, already skinny, is losing weight because she cannot eat. She says she is sick. Someone else will have to cook. She is going back to bed.

I made up those names and situations. Normally about half the names would be spiritual names. The complaints were invented along with the names, but they are fairly typical, though exaggerated for effect. Srinivasan deals with them one at a time, and the scene holds together. Karma Yoga, to be effective, has to start with the leadership. All kinds of individual situations must be overcome for utopia to work. I am surprised by how much good will goes into the work that keeps the ashram going. I have noticed that happy people enjoy working, and I have also seen people become happier by working, even when they did not want to work at first.

Leading by Example

Among other duties, the Karma Yoga of swamis is to set an example. More is expected of them because of the vows they have taken. Swami Padmapananda is the swami in residence at the Yoga Ranch and a South African by birth. He went to Israel to study Hebrew and found vegetarianism and yoga. He has lived at the Yoga Ranch for eight years and has been a swami for almost thirty years. He looks like a large intellectual seabird with a nice smile. His cheerful demeanor, shaved head, and orange robes give him a spiritual air. The personal *sadhana* of a dedicated swami is also Karma Yoga because it creates a spiritual vibration that benefits everyone. The job of a swami is to become a *jivanmukta*. There is a lot of selfless service along the way. Like Srinivasan, Swami Padma is involved in the daily workings of the ashram. The two take turns leading *satsang*s, and they perform *puja*s together like old teammates. Swami Padma, like all the swamis in the organization, is a Hatha Yoga teacher. In baseball terms he is like a utility infielder. He catches a lot of balls. He teaches yoga to the inmates of two nearby prisons. He is a counselor to inmates and maintains a prison outreach program that sends copies of Swami Vishnu-Devananda's *Complete Illustrated Book of Yoga* free of charge to inmates who request it.

A paying guest does not have to make a lot of big choices during the average day at a Sivananda ashram. Handing over control is part of the magic. But you can choose what you want to do for selfless service. You can even choose not to do anything, but that would not be the best choice, for reasons I will explain. The moment of decision comes during brunch, when a staff member with a clipboard passes from table to table, asking all the guests if they have any preference in their Karma Yoga assignments. Brunch provides a captive audience—it is the best time to find everybody in the same place. That makes it the best time to muster the troops for the day's Karma Yoga assignments.

If the ashram is like a body, it follows that all jobs are important. If the organs of elimination are blocked, the brain will quickly cease to care about anything else. Keeping the ashram in working order takes constant attention. When you work for the benefit of others you become a part of that body. You can forget about yourself and shift the focus to the job at hand. I experience this as a release from my individual and

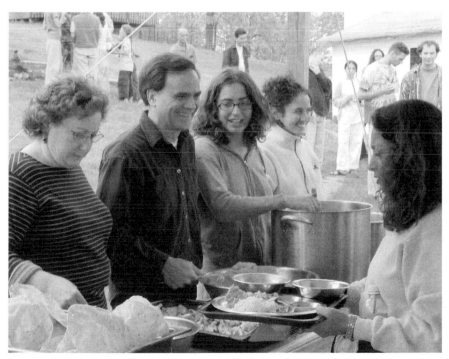

Karma Yoga is an important aspect of ashram life. At the Yoga Ranch, guests are asked to spend an hour each day in selfless service. Here, guests help serve brunch to other guests under the tent that serves as the ashram's dining area in warm weather.

often selfish concerns. I have a friend who experiences a letdown when he comes home from the ashram. Sometimes I do, too. He says he misses the Karma Yoga, the contentment that comes with teamwork and an easy conscience.

A story about the difference between heaven and hell illustrates this point. In heaven and hell, everybody had to wear handcuffs for some reason. Who knows why? Maybe God made a bet with Satan. Bear with me, it gets even worse. All were given spoons with handles much longer than their arms. The tables were laden with good food. What to do? In hell, they starved. They tried to feed themselves, but they went hungry because they couldn't get the food into their mouths. Not only that, but they made a huge mess and spilled food all over the place. In heaven, the situation was completely different. Everybody got plenty to eat, and very little was spilled. Why? In heaven they fed each other. This simple and implausible story has truth in it.

Karma Yoga is like the final relaxation at the end of the *asana* class, the time when you begin to notice the subtle changes that began hours ago when you got out of bed for meditation. Karma Yoga is time to zone out. I experience the difference as a sense of release and oneness with the job at hand. This one-pointed, undivided mind creates a sensation that goes beyond pleasure because it is felt as joy, which combines goodness with pleasure. These are not heroic jobs, but they have to be done. Karma Yoga, the path of selfless service, is the yoga for everybody. The jobs break down into two categories—inside or outside, depending on the weather. Inside jobs are kitchen cleanup, sweeping, vacuuming the dorms, and scrubbing the bathrooms. These are the jobs I have to make myself do at home, but at the ashram I enjoy them. When I scrub a dirty pot I get some of the dirt out of my navel that *asana*s, meditation, and chanting missed.

Outside jobs vary according to the season. When I first started visiting the Ranch, all my jobs were outside. It was spring, and I wanted to be out in the fresh air. I didn't care what I did as long as I was outside. The first Karma yogi I got to know at the Ranch was Bill, a wiry, white-haired Canadian. A former ironworker and biker who took the teacher training about thirty years ago, Bill has essential skills for the mainte-nance of the ashram. If it has to do with building, plumbing, electrical work, landscaping, and all yard work other than gardening, Bill is involved, both in doing and in supervising. He'll get as dirty as the next guy, so you never feel that he's just using you to do something he would not do himself. You never see him doing *asana*s or chanting, but you might catch him in the sauna. Last winter he remodeled it, building new wooden benches, installing new electric lights, and relining the interi-or with fresh cement. He's a good man with a trowel. My first job with Bill was picking up junk and trash from behind the shop and loading it onto a trailer. Then I raked dead leaves from under the porch. Once I sawed off old water pipes with a Saws-All. Another time I threw boul-ders down a hill, where they were used to landscape a wall next to the sauna. In every case I was so inordinately pleased with myself for these little projects that I certainly must have negated some of the good karma I had accrued.

I hate to admit it, but I get satisfaction out of Karma Yoga that is way greater than the exertion I make. "Do you expect anything from your small son, if you do something for him?" asks Swami Sivananda. "In a similar manner, you will have to work for others without expecting any-thing. You will have to expand your heart and think that this whole world is your own Self. It gives you a little pain in the beginning because you never have worked up to this time in this line of selfless, or disin-terested, service. When you have tasted the Bliss of Karma Yoga, you can never leave it."

This seems to be true. Most people seem to welcome a chance to do a simple task dedicated to the greater good. It takes their minds off their own problems. The more complicated the person, the more he or she appreciates something simple to do. Stacking firewood and washing dishes provide a balance to the day's activities. With meditation and *asanas*, the focus is inward. In Karma Yoga, you interact with others. It's like doing a back bend after doing a forward bend. It's designed to make you flexible. The schedule developed by Swami Vishnu-Devananda works the knots out of your back, the hard spots out of your heart, and the soreness out of your head. Some people sink into Karma Yoga effortlessly, like a sponge absorbing water.

Garden work picks up in spring and summer. The garden is managed by Paul, a quiet Irishman with a subtle sense of humor that is mostly expressed through his blue eyes. Paul is well into middle age and had already lived a life on the outside before taking up the ashram. His

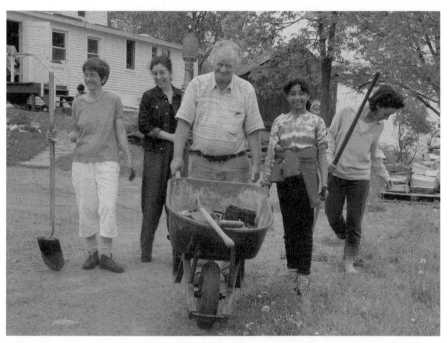

Ashram meals are prepared using the principles of Ayurveda, literally translated as the "science of life." To help achieve a balanced and healthy sattwic diet, some of the food at Yoga Ranch is grown in the ashram's organic garden, where master gardener Paul oversees a team of enthusiastic Karma yogis.

knowledge of organic gardening is deep, and he takes a steady, long-term approach. Paul is in for the long haul and has been at the Yoga Ranch much longer than anyone else. He doesn't say it aloud, but his eyes say, "I've seen 'em come and I've seen 'em go." Like any good gardener, Paul is a patient man, ready to reap what he has sown. Swami Sivananda wrote, "Man sows a seed to attain what he desires to reap. Even so, man does evil deeds and reaps the fruit of pain. He who does virtuous actions reaps good fruits. One reaps fruits according to his Karmas, or actions."

Of course, not everyone who goes to an ashram is a saint. This was never the case. Swami Vishnu-Devananda warned that in India there were people on the run from the law who hid in ashrams. Once he even had to fight a devotee who tried to kill Swami Sivananda with an axe. He succeeded in thwarting the attacker even as the blade descended toward his master's head, barely missing. The next day Swami Sivananda took flowers to his attacker in his jail cell and bowed to him. To this day, eccentric personalities are not shunned in Sivananda ashrams.

The best place to see how an ashram works is the kitchen. I recommend it. The kitchen cleanup at the Ranch is like a modern dance. The performers carry dishes to a steaming sterilizer, remove them, wipe them off, and put them away. The challengers are disorder, dirt, and leftovers. The props are dishcloths, sponges, and mops. The stage is set with a well-blackened, eight-burner Vulcan range at one end, surrounded by cooking pots and knives. The other wall is all about sinks and scullery work. The long wall is dedicated to cleaning, with a stainless steel counter, twin deep sinks, and a spraying area. The hot-water-blasting sterilizer under the counter supplies the music, hissing and churning. It is loaded with dishes and silverware. The dish-laden bins fly into the steaming maw of the sterilizer dirty and emerge sanitary. They come out so fast that two or three human dryers are needed to keep up. The side-by-side deep sinks are for scrubbing pots and pans. That's the leading male role in kitchen cleanup, but women often do it. If you want to be popular at an ashram, take the nastiest jobs but don't shun an easy one. Drying isn't bad. You dry and then put away. There is a sense of closure.

Somebody has to deal with the leftovers. This is a job for an expert, but you might get stuck with it. Leftover food is strangely like karma—a problem for the next meal. It must be incorporated or tossed. This will force you to make some tough decisions about what to keep and what to throw away. In the best of all possible worlds, there would be no leftovers, but inevitably there are. Some are worth saving, and the rest are tossed. As much as possible is composted. There is some big-time Tupperware. After you scrape the pots they go to the sink. The final act is mopping the floor. Then you are done. You go outside. It's a beautiful day. You do not care whether the sky is blue or gray. You have done your duty. You feel good. The sauna beckons.

8

Seven Days in Paradise: A Journal

Look carefully around you and recognize the luminosity of souls.

Sit by those who draw you to that.

—RUMI

Day One: Monday, January 14. The taxi man taking me to Paradise Island is wearing a tie and has a Bible by his side. I find this reassuring. The trip from the airport to Nassau at the other end of New Providence Island takes about forty minutes when there is traffic, and today there is some. Along the way we listen to vigorous radio preaching at a low volume. I suspect it would be louder if I were not there. I am on my way in the blazing Bahama sun to the Sivananda Ashram Yoga Retreat, thinking about yoga in Paradise.

The radio preaching is a sermon all about devotion. In yoga, the path of devotion is called Bhakti Yoga. When we climb to the top of the high-arched bridge to Paradise Island, the radio preacher shouts, "Praise Jesus!" right on cue. It is as if that radio preacher were looking out the windshield at the Atlantis Resort and Hotel looming in the foreground. It is so grand and so pink that it looks like a mirage. There are other

125

hotels, but I don't notice them at first. I know that down there, some-where under a canopy of palm trees, is an ashram, but I can't see it. The noon sun is blinding.

The bridge soars over a busy bay. Great cruise ships belly up to the docks and toot their horns. Nassau's main street is filled with tourists. The Disney ship's horn plays the tune to "Someday My Prince Will Come." Seaplanes glide down from the sky and take off again. Nassau has a real working harbor with lots of docks. The main business is tourism, but there is a commercial fishery and a constant traffic in small freighters. Booze cruises ply the waters regularly along with yachts, fish-ing boats, and jet-skis. The bay has a hustle and bustle that makes Par-adise Island more real. A small amount of fantasy requires a large infrastructure. Meanwhile, down on the island ahead, I see coconut palms like the southwest coast of India. I can see why Swami Vishnu-Devananda would have felt at home in this climate and landscape.

Once off the bridge, we wind on smooth asphalt through green lawns and planned landscaping. James Bond would keep a speedboat in a place like this (in fact, scenes from *Thunderball* were shot nearby). The taxi drops me at the Paradise Island Ferry terminal. A phone call is made, and about twenty minutes later a launch arrives and picks up four of us and takes us to the ashram. There is a hip-looking couple—both pale, so I assume they are from New York—in the boat. A few days later I will meet them again and find out that they are my neighbors in the city. There is a contingent from downtown Manhattan at the ashram. We always find one another wherever we go.

There are no roads to the ashram. My first impression of the ashram from the water is to be charmed by its modesty. It looks like Gilligan's Island in a yogic way. Tall palm trees dominate the view, and the build-ings are tucked into nature. In January the dock still has Christmas ribbons tied to the posts. I feel the ashram vibration, the sense of con-stant spiritual celebration, very strongly. Wherever constant *sadhana* is done, *prana* accumulates. My immediate feeling is that *prana* overflows here; all I have to do is put my cup out and let it be filled. Hand-painted scenes from the Ramayana activate the sides of buildings and make the place feel like a stage set for a celestial drama. There are radiant images of smiling Ganeshas. The elephant-headed one presides at the top of the steps, looking down over the whole ashram, his playground. Christmas lights are everywhere, even though it is daytime. At night they are magical. A Teachers Training Course is under way, and the students fill the temple for the noon lecture on the *Bhagavad Gita* taught by Srinivasan, who has come to the Bahamas to help with the course. The leaders, or *acharya*s, of the Sivananda organization travel to other ashrams to help whenever there is a Teachers Training Course, which is most of the time now, somewhere in the world. More than a hundred students are taking the month-long course, and they bring a lot of energy with them.

The ashram air is fragrant with jasmine and salt. The island light is dazzling. I need to find out where I am staying. I have a huge four-person tent that I borrowed, and now I need a place to set it up. William, the ferryman, takes me around to help me find a spot. This is harder than I expected. I do not notice them at first, but tents are almost edge to edge, tucked into the corners and hidden by vegetation. I see that the tent situation will have to be worked out, so I do the sensible thing and report to the reception area located right smack in the middle of the scene. It looks like a fanciful hot dog stand painted a pale island green, but it is the core of the central nervous system of the community. Important ashram business is done here, including reservations, room assignments, ferry scheduling, mail, telephones, finding people (there is a loudspeaker), and anything else that needs doing. The boss is a good-natured Bahamian woman named Patricia who runs a tight ship. I like the way she can smile while juggling ashram problems. I have one for her—I left a bag behind in the taxi, and all I can remember is that the van was white and the driver wore a tie and had a Bible. "I'll take care of it," she says. Two hours later, I have a room and my bag is in it. It turns out that there are more rooms than tent sites. Meanwhile, Patricia has called all three taxi companies and found my stuff. The nonstop flight from LaGuardia took three hours, and by one o'clock in the afternoon I have a room by the sea with a balcony overlooking the ocean.

The room is part of a tiny house that Srinivasan and Laksmi are using, which Sri has asked me if I wanted to share. Their house has an extra room with a separate entrance. Sri had planned to use the room to do some writing because it had a desk, but he kindly offers it to me. Now I have a lovely room and wonderful neighbors. God is really smiling on me. I was willing to stay in the tent, but this room is perfect— simple and clean. All the linens and the curtains and the rug are shades of white. The familiar small narrow bed tells me that I am at a Sivananda ashram. At six feet, four inches, Sri says that his feet hung over the end. A window runs the length of the wall on the ocean side. There is a framed print of Ram on the wall above the bed. The more I look at these fanciful renditions of Hindu gods, the more they intrigue me. At first I found them off-putting in the extreme, but now I try to read them like books. I once asked Swami Swaroopananda, the director of the ashram on Paradise Island, to explain these images. He said, "They are like maps. The map is not the terrain itself, but it tells you something about the terrain."

After unpacking, I lie on the bed and shut my eyes. After a short nap, it's time for the afternoon yoga class, which is on the bay platform and excellent. The same twelve postures are offered wherever I go; nothing changes, but the class is always different. The teacher is a perky, recently graduated teacher who has stayed on as a Karma yogi. She is still a little nervous, afraid that she will forget something important or make a mistake. She has a nice voice, and sometimes she has to use it to be heard over the boats in the harbor and the wakes washing up under the bay platform. The bay platform classes are noisy, but the sunsets are amazing. Spectacular orange clouds light up the evening sky.

After class I feel as if I deserve a good dinner, and I overeat. I am a fool for buffets. I like everything. Dinner is vegetarian chili, millet and pureed carrot soup, steamed zucchini, and cauliflower. The tossed green salad comes with mung bean sprouts, shredded carrots, and cucumbers. The style is to serve yourself and find a seat at a picnic table in one of the covered pavilions. I sit across from a youngish mother and her teenage daughter, who have come to take the afternoon *asana* class and stayed for dinner. A ferry brought them from the Marriott Hotel. They are glad to get a dinner that is not all about meat, they say, because that was what the others in their party liked. They came to the right place—no meat here. They leave to meet up again with their committed carnivores, and an intense woman in her late twenties from Montreal sits down, saying that she is taking the Teachers Training Course even though she has had only seven months of yoga practice. She is not sure that it is enough. I tell her that it was enough in my experience—that if she tries hard, there will be no problem. She decided at the last minute to take a leave of absence from her Canadian government job and is still in shock about it. She wants to do something important with her time, and she is very determined to stand on her head. I assure her that she will find it easy. Wanting to stand on your head is a sure indication that you will succeed. I like to teach students to do it. The first time people stand on their head, they are so happy. Unless they have a neck injury or a physical problem, they all learn eventually.

The after-dinner drill is utterly familiar. We stand in line to wash our own dishes, using three deep sinks. Then they are sterilized. Now that I have eaten I feel content. Conversations are going on all around me. Conversations begun at the picnic table continue through the dishwashing. I like to talk, but any yogic material that I have ever read about talking says it is a waste of energy. Some yogis practice *mouna*, or self-imposed silence. Even worse than talking is gossiping. Idle hours spent gossiping constitute one of the dangers of ashram life. In the insular ashram world, some people get addicted to gossip. They like their soap operas to have a spiritual backdrop. There is a fine line when conversation turns to gossip. I don't mind hearing gossip, but I feel guilty when I repeat it. I am not sure there is a great ethical difference, but I listen to what people say and I find it interesting, especially since I am writing a book. This instinct to eavesdrop is an advantage at a newspaper—perhaps even a virtue.

Two people across from me are talking about yoga in Israel. She is so beautiful that I have to make myself notice him too. I have a friend who just opened a Sivananda-affiliated center in a resort by the Dead Sea. There is a Sivananda jet set that flies from ashram to ashram. The people in it are not rich, but they manage to stay in motion. Sometimes they stay months at an ashram as Karma yogis, and then they go to some other place. They practice the international style of *sadhana*. This is a Sivananda ashram hallmark. When I go to the Bahamas I see people that I've met in India. The Sivananda circuit includes stops in Canada, or in the Catskills, or Grass Valley, Austria, Paris, Tel Aviv—and these are just a few of the places. The woman says, "There are many affiliated Sivananda centers in Israel. A new one just opened by the Dead Sea." This is a small world. I ask if they have been there, and she says yes. I can't tell whether they are a couple. "I know Ganesha and his new wife, Karuna," I say.

"Yes, he is a great guy," she says. "Sivananda yoga is very popular in Israel."

She is one of the most graceful creatures I have ever seen. Yoga is like a finishing school for posture. Her back has always been straight, but now it is straighter. She has classic Sephardic features and long black hair. To keep the conversation going, I ask about Ganesha. "He is doing well," she says. "The place is very beautiful."

I am always meeting Israelis and British subjects at Sivananda ashrams. Swami Vishnu pulled off some of his most successful peace flights in those countries. The stunts brought a lot of attention to yoga, and that's when he got the nickname Flying Swami. Some serious travelers are to be found at ashrams. My friend Ganesha is living the third act of his life creating his own ashram by the Dead Sea. The way yoga is expanding, I am sure he will succeed. He was in the restaurant business and knows how to please people. It takes a calling for service to have an ashram. I think he has it. Ganesha has a natural way of making people feel special. Swami Sivananda had this trait—each of his disciples thought he was the master's favorite. I am sure that in this life or the next, I will see Ganesha again. Everybody keeps turning up. I am sure I will see this beautiful woman who is washing her dishes again, too, and I look forward to that.

If I squint my eyes, Paradise Island looks a little bit like Kerala, in southern India. If I shut my eyes, the yoga retreat feels like a party waiting to happen. That could be the Teachers Training Course. Most of the students are in their twenties, the age of energy. The brightness of the sun, the blue ocean, the intense green vegetation, and the high spirits are contagious.

Club Med next door and the Atlantis Resort offer the great sun and sea too, but I am happy here. The kind of people who want a yoga vacation are a healthy lot. Just being there feels as if you are doing the right thing. A feeling of idealism and innocence contrasts nicely with the backdrop of a casino. Atlantis makes me feel better about being at the ashram. I am more content, and happy not to be in a place where someone is out to separate me from my money. Not having to gamble is a blessing. I am a terrible gambler. At the ashram there is almost nothing to spend money on—once I am there, everything is included. Enlightenment is thrown in for free.

During evening meditation, the Booze Cruise steams down the channel past the temple, blasting music. In India there was a wildlife refuge across the lake where lions roared day and night. While I was trying to meditate they made noises that sounded as if they were mating. After a while I even got used to that. On Paradise Island it's the Booze Cruise. Like the lions, these high-octane parties keep going way after sunset.

When *satsang* ends, I walk back to my room. The atmosphere is *sattwic*, pure and elevated. I feel the vibe of the room, and it is soothing. I hear the sea lapping the beach. My first day in Paradise is closing. My eyes are heavy after the first day. The hard, narrow bed will do nicely.

Day Two: Tuesday, January 15. I hear the morning bell at 5:30, sounding as if it is just outside my window, but I don't move. Then it sounds as if it is in my head. I have to be dreaming—it is too early for this to be the real bell. I do not get out of bed. When I finally wake up, the sun is shining brightly, and I know then that my mind has played a trick on me. The sleep was delicious, but I suspected I was *tamasic*. Swami Sivananda would not approve. Too much sleep makes a person dull. I don't roar like a lion of Vedanta in my sleep.

My watch says 7:30. That must have been the real bell after all. I have overslept by two hours. The light filtering through the white curtains looks pure and alluring, like *Brahman*. I feel there is something special about this day already. The ocean outside is lapping against the white sand, calling me enticingly. There is just time enough for a swim before *asana* class. I roll out of the sack and put on my swimming trunks. On the ride from the airport to the ashram, I asked the taxi driver to please stop so that I could buy a bathing suit. He stopped, but reluctantly. All the bathing suits I liked cost about fifty dollars, so I bought one I did not like at all for sixteen dollars. It had a lurid sunset-over-palms motif printed on it, and I think it was too small. It was in the bag I left in the taxi. I did not want that bathing suit. The one consolation is that I do not have to look at myself in it. So I suck in my stomach a little and put on my Speedo. If I keep up with yoga, one day I will look good in it again.

The ocean calls me and I answer. Cool salt water wakes me up. To say that it is like being baptized would be accurate. I tingle all over, completely awake now. I do the breaststroke with my eyes open. The bottom looks so close I can almost touch it. I feel blessed to be in the Bahamas in January. I want to see what a week of serious *asana* practice will do. Meanwhile, back in the ocean the only sound I hear is the waves breaking.

I swim straight out to get a look at the ashram from the ocean side. About two hundred yards out, I turn and look back. The ashram seems to retreat to shelter behind the palms. About half a mile down the beach to my left is the Atlantis, looking so enormous and out of scale that it seems to inhabit a world of its own making. Between Atlantis and the ashram is Club Med, making a nice transition between Atlantis and the ashram. It is an adult playground built on a former estate, whose old buildings give it a hint of past grandeur. It has enormous manicured lawns and an international clientele. During the day the beach is home to a flotilla of Hobie Cats and to sunbathers from northern countries who prefer all-over tans. They get out early, before the sun becomes too hot. As I pan to the right I see the walls of private estates. Loads of movie stars and rock stars live and have lived behind those walls. Way off to the right is the lighthouse. I swim back, shower, and dress for class. Clean clothes feel so good. So far everything is perfect—perfect because I feel at one with it.

A lizard watches me from the rail of the balcony as I approach the house. I've seen it before, or one like it, and simply thought, "There is a lizard. I haven't seen one of those in a while." Now I am in one of those exalted states where I feel the tiny creature's nervous energy. It lasts less than a second, but I get a transcendental rush as if I am seeing this lizard as a manifestation of *Brahman*. The universal spirit is there in the quivering tail. This is a heavy little flash. In yogic philosophy, or Vedanta, this *Brahman* is God. I am not saying that I become enlightened or that I see God; I just have a delightful glimpse of the bliss of concentration. It's like the feeling a hack golfer gets after hitting a long drive and it stays in the fairway. The ashram exists to give people a taste of this *Atmic* bliss. An appetite for Self-realization is stoked by little moments like that. A *jivanmukta* (liberated spirit) can live all the time in this exalted state. The *jivanmukta* sees *Brahman* everywhere. The ashram streamlines my life so that I do not have any worries, and that is very important. In subtle ways, all the *sadhana* that has been practiced at the ashram supports me. The ashram to me is a playground, an Eden, and a second chance. It always welcomes me with open arms. The second day is when the good feeling kicks in strongly.

The salt water leaves an antiseptic tingle. The *asana* platform is painted zinc yellow and bright blue—one of those color combinations that works only in the Caribbean. There is plenty of room for sixty students. The Atlantic Ocean is the big presence. There are some fairly amazing bodies among the students, and some of the more adept of them do elaborate warm-ups. I can't wait for the class. I roll out my purple sticky mat in a shady spot under the branches of a pine tree. I know that this is my spot. The sound of my thoughts is washed away by the waves. Concentrating on the flow of breath is the surest way to calmness. As the breathing becomes softer and subtler my brain gets a rest. I scan my body for any tension or pain. My right shoulder hurts in the joint, and my back is stiff from too much sleep. I guide my breath to these areas, and they relax. What I am really moving is *prana*, or energy. It is supposed to respond to mental commands and go where I ask it to go. I send as much *prana* as I can to my sore shoulder and back. As I inhale, I say silently to myself, "I am breathing energy into my shoulder." As I exhale I say to myself, "I am exhaling the pain." It sounds corny, but it works. After two or three directed breaths, the shoulder is better, free enough to stretch fully overhead. I still know the soreness is there, but I can work with it.

At eight the sun is up, but still behind the palms. We do the Sun Salutation. My breath and movement are smooth and together. I surrender control to the teacher, Laksmi, and just follow instructions. As

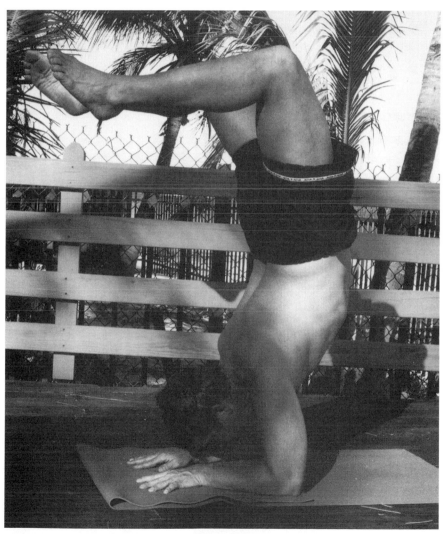

Regular asana *practice will help improve strength, flexibility, and posture. Here, the author practices his version of the Scorpion Pose during an* asana *class at the Sivananda Ashram Yoga Retreat in the Bahamas.*

each posture comes along she guides us expertly into position. To know how to verbalize inner movements, the teacher needs to know the posture from the inside out, and she does. We move from *asana* to *asana*. The class passes like a dream, one *asana* at a time. During final relaxation my mind wanders toward the kitchen about fifty feet away. I can smell the fresh bread baking. My stomach grumbles during the final chant.

There is no need to ring a bell announcing brunch. People just seem to know when it's time to eat. We need to exercise restraint, because the food is tasty and we can have all we want. A large stainless steel bowl of oatmeal and another big bowl of granola are the starters. Except for the sliced oranges, these are the only choices that most people would consider normal breakfast food. There are no eggs, but there is plenty of broccoli, baked tofu, and tossed green salad with fixings such as sunflower seeds and shredded carrots. I see some healthy appetites. The plates are often piled quite high with food in the morning. This makes it less embarrassing for me. Mortification of the flesh will not be necessary either. The food is impressive and very fresh. The home-baked bread could be rated as addictive. Losing weight here will have to be a conscious act.

Day Three: Wednesday, January 16. At two o'clock, Swami Swaroopananda is lecturing on the philosophy of yoga for the students taking the Teachers Training Course. Guests can attend the daily lectures; there is always room at the back. Every day except Sunday the students must attend a two-hour talk on the philosophy of yoga. At noon there is a mandatory one-hour lecture on the *Bhagavad Gita*. The students are like sponges that can't absorb any more water. Some of them are dazed. They have so much yoga poured into them that it will take years to absorb. To break new ground in the mind is exhausting.

The lecture is held in the temple, a building so close to the ground that tall people have to duck when they come in the front door. From outside it looks like a large, ordinary shed. It was doubtless a shed before it was a temple—if you were starting from scratch you would never think to build such a temple. The only sign that it is a temple is the line of sandals outside the door. It looks just as much like a good place to build a boat as a good place to hear a lecture on Vedanta.

I get there late and sit all the way in the back with the students who are Vedanta-impaired. The back row is just the way it was in my Teachers Training Course in India. The students braid each other's hair, doodle, and try to act as if they are awake. Every once in a while, someone looks up and asks, "What did he say?"

Swami Swaroopananda has a reputation as a Vedantist, and I am excited about attending his lecture. He makes the subject come alive. He has the speech cadence of a rabbi, and his turn of phrase is well suited to the subject. He carries ideas lightly to their conclusion with a crushing logic. The source of today's lecture is an astonishingly bold statement on the nature of reality by the seventh-century nondualist philosopher Adi Shankaracharya, who said, "Brahman is real. The universe is unreal. Brahman and *Atman* are One." There is something almost surreal about this assertion. Who can say "The universe is unreal" and really mean it? Since the universe is always changing, Shankaracharya reasoned that it could not be real. Because *Brahman* is unchanging, he considered it real. Further, he said that the human soul, *Atman,* is the same as *Brahman.* If you think about things like this for a long time you may become a Jnana yogi—a thinking personality. I can tell that Swami Swaroopananda is into the subject.

"What are *upadhis*?" Swami Swaroopananda looks around the temple for a brave soul to answer the question. He finds no takers and answers himself: "*Upadhi*s are that which veils the consciousness. They are also called limiting adjuncts. *Upadhi*s create the illusion of limitation even when there is no such thing. *Maya,* the cosmic drama, manifests itself in the individual as *avidya*, or ignorance. This *avidya* makes us forget that we are God, and we identify with the body and the mind, though we are neither body nor mind. Our true nature is *Atman*. When the Self identifies with the *upadhis*, it is called *jiva*."

Swami Swaroopananda has taught this course many times. He knows that much of the information will not get through to the students the first time around, but he acts with the assurance that something does stick. His approach is nicely balanced between playful and serious to hold the interest of the class. The keen students sit in the front, where paying attention is easier. Some students are much less interested in philosophy than others, and they sit in the back, where they are unlikely to be asked any questions. Swami Swaroopananda asks, "What is the meaning of *Sat-chid-ananda*?" and the student on the floor in front of me wakes up, surprising me because he had seemed to be down for the count. He whispers loudly, "What's he talking about?" Someone up front says, "Existence, Knowledge, and Bliss Absolute." When he hears this, he says, "Oh," and goes back to sleep.

In my training course in India, where it gets hot, fatigue would set in by early afternoon when the really heavy information came in bucket loads. Swami Mahadevananda kept students from falling asleep in philosophy class by walking around. Maybe he kept himself from falling asleep, too. The subject of *advaita* Vedanta overwhelms people when they first hear about it. Students do not fall asleep because the subject is dull; they fall asleep when their brains fill up.

Swami Swaroop keeps a cheerful countenance in the midst of the confusion. "There are 33,000,000 names for gods," he asserts with relish. "This means there are this many aspects of *Ishwara*. What is *Ishwara*?" He does not wait for an answer. "*Ishwara* is *Brahman* in association with *Maya*. *Ishwara* is God with attributes. When *Brahman* is manifest, it is called *Ishwara*, or the personal God. You can relate to *Ishwara*. In other words, the names are many, but God is one."

Finally he tells a story about how not to misunderstand the guru. "Adi Shankaracharya is walking through the town followed by his disciples. It's a hot, dry, dusty day. He goes into a bar and orders a beer, and the disciples follow his example. They think it's okay if the teacher is doing it. So they are all drinking beer, having a good time. After they finish the beer, Shankaracharya takes them back out to the street, and they follow him. They walk to a blacksmith shop, and Shankaracharya goes inside and picks up a cup of molten iron from the fire, drinks some, and offers the rest for his disciples to drink. But none of them want any. The moral of this story is, don't imitate the teacher. Teachers do strange things." I wonder what Shankaracharya would have done if a disciple had drunk the iron. The guru relationship is the source of many cautionary tales.

At the end of the class, I go up front to where some of the students and senior staff members have gathered around to settle questions that came up in the lecture. One question was "Why do we have to suffer?" While he admits that suffering is an illusion, Swami Swaroopananda asserts, "The experience of suffering has a place in creation. You can never realize yourself in heaven because there is no suffering there. That is why it is so important to have a human birth. Suffering is the antiseptic of the soul. Suffering is required to see what is behind creation." He uses another example. "If you want to have a fire, first you need friction. Then you get a flame. Then you get light. Suffering is a part of creation. Welcome to creation. Why are these knocks of life coming? To wake you up! If there is no pain, there is no reason to do anything. You can be a potato. Mental anguish tells you that mental balance must be reestablished. Who are you? You are God forgetting you are God. Until you remember that, you will suffer. Buddha said suffering is not knowing your real nature."

The swami asks one last question. "Why did God create freedom of choice? Because without it everything is unreal. Don't blame God.

You are blaming yourself. The first ignorance is when you think you are separate from God." Folding his hands enigmatically, he adds, "Silence is not what we think silence is."

Day Four: Thursday, January 17. At brunch today I spill my bowl of granola on the picnic table as I sit down. Luckily, there is no milk in it yet. I wipe up the mess and laugh at my clumsiness. This yoga sure helps me lighten up. Across the table, an emphatic Englishwoman is telling a Sri Lankan man something about *Moby-Dick*. I interrupt their conversation with my granola incident. We introduce ourselves. Linda is a milliner and has a hat shop in Manhattan's artsy SoHo district. She has the dramatic flair of a person who could make a living selling hats. The angular Sri Lankan, Methun, looks serious but bemused. He is a professor of molecular biology. He asks about me, and I tell him I am writing a book about a week in an ashram.

Moby-Dick, with the obsessive Ahab and its whaling lore, is one of my favorite books. It is so full of passion. I could not imagine reading it at the yoga retreat, but Linda, the literary milliner, says she is enjoying it, especially when Ahab comes out on deck and fits his ivory peg-leg into holes bored into the quarterdeck. I ask if she has gotten to the part where Melville digresses on whiteness, the eeriness inherent in white.

"No, not yet," she says.

Then another new person, Lisa, shows up at the picnic table with her boyfriend, Wolfgang. We arrived on the same Delta flight. They sit down with their trays. As it turns out, Lisa is a friend of Linda's and also a milliner. Lisa's hat shop is on Mulberry Street in trendy Nolita, which used to be Little Italy but now is an area of cute boutiques. Wolfgang does something with computers. He has short dark hair and speaks English with a bit of German in his accent. He has very little hair, and she has a lot. They both wear straw hats she designed. They look good together, hats and all. Lisa takes an interest in my book project and asks a tough question.

"What is the conflict?" she asks. "For a story to be interesting it has to have a conflict."

She has a point. Where is my maniacal Ahab? Where is my inscrutable Moby-Dick? "The conflict is in me," I say, "between my higher and lower natures. It is a titanic struggle." It sounds tongue in cheek, but it sounds true. So far I have no conflict with the ashram. There are no people who are getting on my nerves. I have crossed over into the ecstatic phase. Now I have met all my New York neighbors. They are an interesting group.

"Did anyone ever call you the Mad Hatters?" I ask, thinking I am so clever.

"They do it all the time," says Lisa.

"Then I won't," I say.

Day Five: Friday, January 18. Today is going to be a great *asana* day. I have been building up to this. I feel it coming. I jump out of bed at first bell, put on bathing trunks, and dive into the dark ocean, surrounded by stars. The saltiness of it purifies my outer layer. I roll over on my back and look up into the charcoal tropical sky. There is still no hint of dawn. I get out and shower in the electric light. I am starting to get some serious contentment from *sattwa* in the Bahamas. All the Hatha Yoga is starting to pay off. I dry off and get dressed for *satsang*. Subtle changes are starting to happen. I get to the temple early and put my mat down to the right of the altar. My back is already stronger and more flexible. I am sitting straighter with less effort. I close my eyes and listen to my thoughts as I adjust my posture. I feel a shift in the awareness of my body, a distance. The mantra begins to regulate my breathing. When my mind wanders I bring it back. When the half hour is up, my foot feels strange to touch, like a piece of meat. But the meditation was good. I rub the foot and it comes back to life.

Asana class is excellent. Toward the end I feel totally energized and have a breakthrough. I can do the Peacock Pose for the first time. I never thought I would be able to hold my body straight like a plank and balance on my palms, but to my amazement I did. I was so surprised I did it twice to make sure. The benefits of *Mayurasana* are described in *Hatha Yoga Pradipika,* which says, "This *asana* cures diseases of the stomach, glands, and spleen, and removes all diseases caused by an excess of wind, bile, and phlegm. It easily digests food taken immoderately and promiscuously, and reduces to ashes even the terrible poison halahala." Whatever that is.

I am meeting Brother Rolph Fernandes for brunch. He is a Franciscan monk who has spent many years in India. He has agreed to talk to me about chanting. I met him at dinner the night before, and I was taken by his understanding of the relationships between religions. I race to get there on time, but he is waiting. We get our food and sit down. There is too much noise, so we find a couple of chairs in the yard. I ask him about the problem that people from other faiths have with chanting.

"The ashram is not a Western idea," he says. "When you go there you must expect that things are going to be different. It's not like going to McDonald's. I would tell people to look at it as a learning experience. Be open from the very beginning. When ashrams started in India, there would be a holy man and people would come to hear his teaching and they would build huts nearby and then they had a spiritual community. It stands to follow," he says, "that if an ashram is founded by someone, any religion that is taught there would reflect these beliefs. In a Sivananda ashram, it is Vedanta that is going to be taught. It's a good thing to be exposed to this, to see what our beliefs have in common. People should know the rules ahead of time. When you take off your shoes, take all your Western prejudices off and leave them outside of the temple with your shoes.

"Swami Vishnu-Devananda was a man of God, and he was a Hindu. They get up in the morning and meditate and they chant. When you come to an ashram, that is what you do. Nobody obliges you to sing along. Chanting is harder than taking off your shoes. The only advice I can give is that it is something that each person has to work out for themselves. I have to ask how far I am prepared to go to think of God under a different name than the one my tradition has taught me to use. The Vedas existed before the Bible was written. If they have existed so long it is because God has allowed it. Maybe He wants to teach us something from this tradition."

Day Six: Saturday, January 19. Today is to be a vacation from the yoga vacation. So far I have not missed an *asana* class or a *satsang*. Today I plan to do both and see Nassau. The plan is hatched at brunch. The downtown brunch crowd keeps growing. Now it also includes Ananda, also known as Paul, a programmer who teaches at the center in New York; Wendy, a marketing person; Sarah, an actress from Los Angeles; and Allison, a yoga teacher. Anybody can join—you just have to show up. I ask if anyone is ready to go to Nassau, and Linda says she wants to go.

We catch the ferry across the bay and are entertained by a tour guide. His patter begins when the ferry pulls away from the dock. "The first attraction is the Atlantis Resort Casino, which was backed financially by Michael Jackson and the Queen of England. Now you see a villa that was used in the movie *Thunderball*. Next are Club Med and the Yoga Retreat. They call *it* Club Meditation. You can go there and take yoga classes if you want to, but there are four rules that you have to follow. The first one is you don't eat any meat. The second rule is no cigarettes. The third rule is no alcohol, and the fourth is no hanky panky. I can live with the first two rules but not the last two." He says other things, too, but these are the most appropriate.

We get off the ferry and walk down the main street of town. Linda is an adventurous traveler and storyteller who does accents very well, especially Indian accents. She is telling stories of a trip she and Lisa made to India. We get off the main street, which is lined with fancy shops near the cruise ship dock, and sit down in a café. I order a beer, feeling positively delinquent, and Linda has white wine. We are on a mission to find the fish-fry restaurants at the end of town, which are supposed to be the best places in Nassau. Along the way we do a nice amount of sightseeing.

Nassau's British colonial history is well represented in the library. This three-story, eight-sided colonial building had once been the prison, with a real dungeon. Upstairs there are skulls of Arawak Indians among old unlabeled exhibits of shells and old photos. An attempt at making it a museum faded. Each floor has a balcony all the way around. The library is in a square planted with tall palm trees behind the courthouse. During an English crackdown on brigands, several pirates were held there and executed. All day I feel as if I was skipping school, especially at the library.

Our fish-fry mission takes us on a long bayside walk where there are signs of genuine Bahamian life. Here the tourists are a minority. About a mile from downtown on the bay is a cluster of restaurants filled with local people. This has to be the place. I have a conch salad, which is like a ceviche, and Linda has fried conch. Anyone who likes seafood would be happy here. I decide that I like the local beer, which is called Kalik. Linda is a tireless sightseeing partner—and fun to eat with, too. A woman who likes to eat makes a good partner at dinner. She is taller than I and can give me a run for my money in the appetite department. We find the real flavor of the Bahamas at the restaurant. It's a good thing we have eaten well, because the walk back takes us on a winding path. Hours later we cross the bridge back to Paradise Island. The sun is setting. This time I can spot the ashram. Now it feels like home.

Day Seven: Sunday, January 20. The bed is feeling great when the bell rings for meditation. I am glad not to be leaving the ashram today. My week is coming to an end, and this is my last full day. I start to feel a little sad that it is ending. Everything is the same, but it feels so different. After a week the ashram has become like home. I have made the adjustment. At *satsang* I meditate with better attention and chant with a little more feeling. I hear the words of the swami with more understanding. I let myself fall into the present and stay there as long as possible. The morning *asana* class is held on the platform by the ocean. I take my place under the pine and watch the needles fall all around me during relaxation. My breathing connects with the waves, and I feel peaceful. During the entire class I keep the awareness of my breath and feel strong and peaceful. In every posture my breath holds me steady. After a week of intense practice, I can feel the transformation from the inside. My shoulder is healthy again after months of soreness. My lower back is not stiff in the morning. Once I got to a certain age I felt that my body had changed forever, but a week in an ashram has proved to me that I can be better than before. This is not a matter of turning back the clock—I am really getting closer to what I already am. Progress in Hatha Yoga is measurable in every posture. By doing the same twelve poses in each class, I can gauge the differences for the whole body. Incremental changes add up. I start to understand how to use the breath when I practice twice a day. The breath starts to set me free.

The downtown brunch group now spills across two picnic tables. There are so many people who live near one another in the city that we make plans to have a reunion a week after we get back. Telephone numbers and e-mail addresses are exchanged. I look around the table and see happiness in all the faces around me. They have gone through the same changes. Maybe this was an extraordinary week and this was a special group, but the energy is shooting out all over the place. We are all in high spirits because Krishna Das will be performing at evening *satsang*.

The day passes quickly, with a long swim in the ocean and another class of *asanas*. After dinner, the temple starts to fill up early. I stake out a spot up close, but off to the side. Thirty minutes of meditation seems to take only five. To say that Krishna Das is eagerly anticipated would be an understatement. Among yogis who practice Bhakti Yoga, Krishna Das is famous. I have only heard his chanting on CDs, but they remind me of my Teachers Training Course in India. On a bus trip to temples in the south, his chants on the tape player melted into the landscape, and it felt like a sacred party. He reminds me of India, but he is an American who found his guru, Neem Karoli Baba, in India. He carried his devotion in his heart.

We skip the Sunday chants and cut straight to Krishna Das, who takes the stage with his tabla player. He wears wire-rimmed glasses and a black T-shirt and has short gray hair. He has the look of an East Village hipster as he fiddles around with his amplifier. The tabla play-

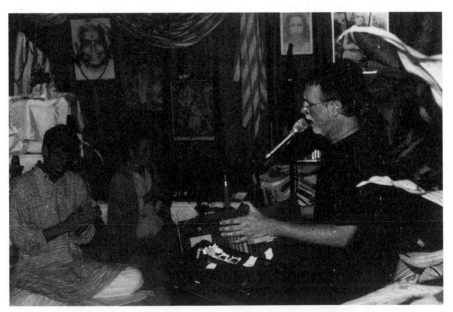

The famous kirtan singer Krishna Das leads the chanting in the temple at the Bahama Yoga Retreat. Krishna Das's devotional chanting mesmerizes audiences worldwide, inspiring people to clap their hands or get up and dance.

er tunes his drum, and the excitement builds. Krishna Das has charisma, but he plays it down. He introduces himself and his drummer and tells some stories. Then he looks around the room and says, "I never wanted to chant so much. All I wanted to do all day was to sit around and look at my guru. That was it. I was completely satisfied. All I wanted to do was sit there and look at him. One day Swamiji asked a disciple if she wanted to see God. She said, 'Oh no, Swamiji, I have to catch a bus so that I can get home on time to cook for the family.'"

He looks for his throat lozenges and finds that ants have gotten them. He fusses around with the wrapper, looks up, and says, "You people are lucky. You like to sing. In India there were about twenty *kirtan-wallahs* who did all the chanting for Mahara-ji, until one day one of them came on to one of the Western women. When Mahara-ji saw this, he packed them all up on a bus and sent them away. So with all the *kirtan-wallahs* gone, who was going to lead the chanting? The Westerners. So we were up on stage with Mahara-ji, but we couldn't see him. This should have been heaven, right? We were in the Himalayas chanting Hare Raama, Hare Raama, Raama Raama, Hare Hare, Hare Krishna, Hare Krishna, Krishna Krishna, Hare Hare, all day. Let me tell you—it wasn't heaven. It was boring. Sometimes I would think about my girlfriend and all kinds of things, and I'd get excited and chant HARE KRISHNA! HARE KRISHNA! Then I would think about how she left me and I'd chant hare krishna, hare krishna. Sometimes I would be feeling good and sometimes I would be feeling bad. I was getting tired of chanting the same thing day after day. Then I realized that whatever I was feeling, the chant was still there."

When he chants the Mahamantra Meltdown, it seems to lift the roof off the temple. It is pure bliss. He sings the lead, and we sing the response. This is what making a joyful noise unto the Lord is all about. The air is charged with *prana*. The feeling touches each person and grows stronger. The chant continues for about ten minutes. At the end I know what Bhakti Yoga is all about. Some people go into a trance, and some have to dance. The chants keep coming, and the feeling keeps growing. Krishna Das paces the concert with stories between chants. He is really funny, and the laughter helps open our hearts. We need the stories to come down, and when the next chant comes, we are galvanized once more. The sound is celestial, and the air is thick with *Shakti.*

When the concert ends we all chant "Om," and for a moment there is silence. Then a party boat blasts "A Little Bit of Monica" to bring us back into the "real" world. Krishna Das smiles at that and says, "It's just like India: *kirtan* wherever you go."

A Directory of Ashrams

Within North America
Sivananda Ashram Yoga Farm
14651 Ballantree Ln., Comp. 8
Grass Valley, CA 95949
(530) 272-9322
Fax: (530) 477-6054
YogaFarm@sivananda.org

The Expanding Light Retreat: Ananda's Retreat Center
14618 Tyler Foote Rd.
Nevada City, CA 95959
(800) 346-5350
info@expandinglight.org
www.expandinglight.org

Mount Madonna Center
445 Summit Rd.
Watsonville, CA 95076
(408) 847-0406
Fax: (408) 847-2683
programs@mountmadonna.org

Kashi Ashram
11155 Roseland Rd.
Sebastian, FL 32950
(800) 226-1008
email-kashinfo@kashi.org

Kripalu Center
P.O. Box 793
West Street, Route 183
Lenox, MA 01240
(800) 741-7353
(413) 448-3152
request@kripalu.org

Omega Institute
150 Lake Dr.
Rhinebeck, NY 12572
(800) 944-1001
registration@eomega.org

Shree Muktananda Ashram
SYDA Foundation
371 Brickman Rd.
P.O. Box 600
South Fallsburg, NY 12779-0600
(845) 434-2000
www.siddhayoga.org

Sivananda Ashram Yoga Ranch Colony
P.O. Box 195
Budd Rd.
Woodbourne, NY 12788
(845) 436-6493
Fax: (845) 434-1032
YogaRanch@sivananda.org

Himalayan International Institute of Yoga Science and Philosophy
RR 1, Box 1127
Honesdale, PA 18431
(570) 253-5551
(800) 822-4547
info@Himalayaninstitute.org
www.Himalayaninstitute.org

Satchidananda Ashram—Yogaville
Route 1, Box 1720
Buckingham, VA 23921
(434) 969-3121
iyi@yogaville.org
www.yogaville.org

Yasodhara Ashram
Box 9
Kootenay Bay, British Columbia
Canada V0B 1X0
(800) 661-8711
Fax: (250) 227-9494
yashram@netidea.com

Sivananda Ashram Yoga Camp
673 8th Ave.
Val Morin, Quebec
Canada J0T 2R0
(819) 322-3226
Fax: (819) 322-5876
HQ@sivananda.org

Outside North America
Sivananda Yoga Retreat House
Am Bichlach Weg 40A
A-6370 Reith bei Kitzbühel, Austria
43-5356-67-404
Fax: 43-5356-67-405
Tyrol@sivananda.org

Sivananda Ashram Yoga Retreat
P.O. Box N7550
Paradise Island, Nassau, Bahamas
(242) 363-2902
Fax: (242) 363-3783
Nassau@sivananda.org

Chateau du Yoga Sivananda
26 Impasse du Bignon
45170 Neuville aux Bois, France
33-2-38-91-88-82

Sivananda Kutir
P.O. Netala, Uttara Kashi Dt.
U.P. Himalayas 249 193, India
01374-22624

Sivananda Yoga Vedanta Dhanwantari Ashram
P.O. Neyyar Dam, Thiruvananthapuram Dt.
Kerala, 695 576, India
0471-273-093
Fax: 0471-272-093
YogaIndia@sivananda.org

Recommended Reading

Bhagavad Gita: Annotated and Explained. Translated by Swami Shri Purohit and annotated by Kendra Crossen Burroughs. Woodstock, Vt.:
   SkyLight Paths Publishing, 2001.

Devi, Yamuna. *Lord Krisha's Cuisine: The Art of Indian Vegetarian Cooking.* New York: Dutton, 1999.

Frawley, David. *Ayurveda and the Mind: The Healing of Consciousness.* Twin
   Lakes, Wis.: Lotus Press, 1997.

Iyengar, B. K. S. *The Tree of Yoga.* Boston: Shambhala, 1989.

Patanjali's Yogasutras: An Introduction. Translation and commentary by
   T. K. V. Desikachar. New Delhi: Affiliated East-West Press in association with Rupa & Col, 1987.

Prabhavananda, Swami. *How to Know God: The Yoga Aphorisms of Patanjali.*
   Translated by Christopher Isherwood. Hollywood, Calif.: Vedanta
   Press, 1996.

Selections from the Gospel of Sri Ramakrishna: Annotated and Explained.
   Translated by Swami Nikhilananda and annotated by Kendra
   Crossen Burroughs. Woodstock, Vt.: SkyLight Paths Publishing, 2002.

Sivananda, Swami. *Bhagavad Gita.* Rishikesh, India: Divine Life Society,
   1995.

———. *Bliss Divine*. Rishikesh, India: Divine Life Society, 1997.

———. *Kundalini Yoga*. Rishikesh, India: Divine Life Society, n.d.

———. *The Practice of Karma Yoga*. Rishikesh, India: Divine Life Society, 1995.

———. *Sadhana*. Rishikesh, India: Divine Life Society, 1998.

Sivananda Yoga Vedanta Center. *The Yoga Cookbook: Vegetarian Food for Body and Mind—Recipes from the Sivananda Yoga Vedanta Centers*. New York: Fireside, 1999.

———. *Yoga Mind and Body (DK Living)*. London and New York: Dorling Kindersley, 1998.

Vivekananda, Swami. *Raja Yoga*. Mayavati, Champawat, Himalayas: Advaita Ashrama, 2000.

Vishnu-Devananda, Swami. *Complete Illustrated Book of Yoga*. New York: Crown, 1995.

———. *Meditation and Mantras*. London: Om Lotus Publishing, 2000.

———. *Hatha Yoga Pradipika*. London: Om Lotus Publishing, 1999.

Glossary

Acharya: Spiritual guide.

Agami karma: Karma that is being created now to be enjoyed later.

Agni: Fire.

Ahimsa: Noninjury to any living thing by thought, word, or deed.

Asana: Posture or pose for controlling the mind and/or body.

Astanga: Eight-limbed, as in the eightfold path of Raja Yoga.

Asteya: Noncovetousness, one of the *yamas*, or restraints, of Raja Yoga.

Atman: The individual soul; the immortal Self.

Avidya: Ignorance; spiritual blindness.

Ayurveda: Holistic system of medicine indigenous to India.

Bhakti: Path of devotion.

Bhava: Attitude of devotion.

Bramacharya: Controlling the sexual energy; one of the *yamas* of Raja Yoga.

Brahmamuhurta: Early morning when night is turning to day; the best time for meditation.

Chakra: One of seven astral centers located in the *shushumna nadi*.

Chitta: Subconscious mind; mind stuff.

Dharana: State of concentration; sixth limb of Raja Yoga.

Dhyana: State of meditation; seventh limb of Raja Yoga.

Guna: One of the three qualities of nature: *sattwa, rajas,* and *tamas.*

Guru: Spiritual teacher; remover of darkness.

Hatha Yoga: The path of yoga giving first attention to the physical body.

Ishwara-pranidhana: Surrender of the ego; one of the *niyama*s of Raja Yoga.

Jiva: Individual soul with ego.

Jivanmukta: Liberated soul in a living person.

Jnana Yoga: Path of knowledge.

Karma: Law of cause and effect, action and reaction.

Karma Yoga: The path of service.

Kirtan: Singing the name of the Lord.

Kriya: Cleansing or purifying exercise.

Kundalini: Cosmic energy, primordial serpent power located in the lower spine.

Mahasamadhi: Final emancipation from the body.

Maya: Illusion, the cosmic drama.

Nada Yoga: The yoga of sound.

Niyama: Religious observances; second limb of Raja Yoga.

Pandit: Scholar of Sanskrit religious texts.

Prana: Vital force; energy.

Pranayama: Controlling the prana; fourth limb of Raja Yoga.

Prarabdha karma: Karma meant to be worked out in this lifetime.

Prasad: Blessed food.

Pratyahara: Withdrawal of energy from the senses.

Puja: Worship.

Raja Yoga: The royal path of yoga; the eight-limbed path laid out by Patanjali.

Rajasic: Active; passionate.

Rishis: Sages.

Sadhana: Spiritual practice.

Samadhi: Superconscious state.

Samskara: A mental impression; behavioral pattern.

Samyama: Perfect restraint, concentration, meditation, and *samadhi*.

Sanchita karma: Stored-up karma.

Sannyasin: A renunciate; a monk.

Sannyasa: Renunciation of social ties.

Santosha: Contentment; one of the *niyamas* of Raja Yoga.

Sat-chid-ananda: Existence, Knowledge, and Bliss Absolute.

Satsang: Company of the wise; association of spiritually minded people.

Sattwic: Pure.

Satya: Truthfulness; one of the *yamas* of Raja Yoga.

Saucha: Purity inside and out.

Shakti: Goddess energy; female power.

Shaktipat: Activation of *Shakti*.

Shushumna nadi: Central *nadi* connecting *chakras*, or astral centers.

Siddhis: Psychic powers.

Sri: Title of respect.

Swami: *Sannyasin*; a monk.

Swamiji: Respectful way of addressing a swami.

Swadhyaya: Study of scriptures.

Tamasic: Impure, dark, or inert.

Tapas: Austerity; one of the *niyamas* of Raja Yoga.

Upadhi: Limiting adjunct.

Vedanta: The philosophy of oneness.

Vritti: Thought wave.

Yama: Ethics; the first limb of Raja Yoga.

Yatra: A pilgrimage to Hindu religious sites.

Yoga: Union with the higher Self.

Notes

Notes

Notes

Notes

Notes

About SKYLIGHT PATHS Publishing

SkyLight Paths Publishing is creating a place where people of different spiritual traditions come together for challenge and inspiration, a place where we can help each other understand the mystery that lies at the heart of our existence.

Through spirituality, our religious beliefs are increasingly becoming a part of our lives—rather than *apart* from our lives. While many of us may be more interested than ever in spiritual growth, we may be less firmly planted in traditional religion. Yet, we do want to deepen our relationship to the sacred, to learn from our own as well as from other faith traditions, and to practice in new ways.

SkyLight Paths sees both believers and seekers as a community that increasingly transcends traditional boundaries of religion and denomination—people wanting to learn from each other, *walking together, finding the way.*

We at SkyLight Paths take great care to produce beautiful books that present meaningful spiritual content in a form that reflects the art of making high quality books. Therefore, we want to acknowledge those who contributed to the production of this book.

PRODUCTION
Tim Holtz, Martha McKinney & Bridgett Taylor

EDITORIAL
Amanda Dupuis, Polly Short Mahoney,
Lauren Seidman & Emily Wichland

COVER DESIGN
Bronwen Battaglia, Scituate, Massachusetts

TEXT DESIGN
Chelsea Cloeter, Scotia, New York

PRINTING & BINDING
Lake Book, Melrose Park, Illinois

Other Interesting Books—Spirituality

Lighting the Lamp of Wisdom: *A Week Inside a Yoga Ashram*
by *John Ittner;* Foreword by *Dr. David Frawley*

This insider's guide to Hindu spiritual life takes you into a typical week of retreat inside a yoga ashram to demystify the experience and show you what to expect from your own visit. Includes a discussion of worship services, meditation and yoga classes, chanting and music, work practice, and more.

6 x 9, 224 pp, b/w photographs, Quality PB, ISBN 1-893361-52-7 **$15.95**;
HC, ISBN 1-893361-37-3 **$24.95**

Waking Up: *A Week Inside a Zen Monastery*
by *Jack Maguire;* Foreword by *John Daido Loori, Roshi*

An essential guide to what it's like to spend a week inside a Zen Buddhist monastery.
6 x 9, 224 pp, b/w photographs, HC, ISBN 1-893361-13-6 **$21.95**

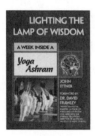 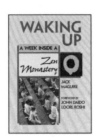 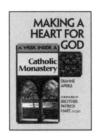 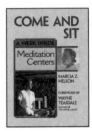

Making a Heart for God: *A Week Inside a Catholic Monastery*
by *Dianne Aprile;* Foreword by *Brother Patrick Hart,* OCSO

This essential guide to experiencing life in a Catholic monastery takes you to the Abbey of Gethsemani—the Trappist monastery in Kentucky that was home to author Thomas Merton—to explore the details. "More balanced and informative than the popular *The Cloister Walk* by Kathleen Norris." *—Choice: Current Reviews for Academic Libraries*

6 x 9, 224 pp, b/w photographs, Quality PB, ISBN 1-893361-49-7 **$16.95**;
HC, ISBN 1-893361-14-4 **$21.95**

Come and Sit: *A Week Inside Meditation Centers*
by *Marcia Z. Nelson;* Foreword by *Wayne Teasdale*

The insider's guide to meditation in a variety of different spiritual traditions. Traveling through Buddhist, Hindu, Christian, Jewish, and Sufi traditions, this essential guide takes you to different meditation centers to meet the teachers and students and learn about the practices, demystifying the meditation experience.

6 x 9, 224 pp, b/w photographs, Quality PB, ISBN 1-893361-35-7 **$16.95**

Or phone, fax, mail or e-mail to: SKYLIGHT PATHS Publishing
Sunset Farm Offices, Route 4 • P.O. Box 237 • Woodstock, Vermont 05091
Tel: (802) 457-4000   Fax: (802) 457-4004   www.skylightpaths.com
Credit card orders: (800) 962-4544 (9AM–5PM ET Monday–Friday)
Generous discounts on quantity orders. SATISFACTION GUARANTEED. Prices subject to change.

Spirituality

Who Is My God?
An Innovative Guide to Finding Your Spiritual Identity
Created by *the Editors at SkyLight Paths*

Spiritual Type™ + Tradition Indicator = Spiritual Identity

Your Spiritual Identity is an undeniable part of who you are—whether you've thought much about it or not. This dynamic resource provides a helpful framework to begin or deepen your spiritual growth. Start by taking the unique Spiritual Identity Self-Test™; tabulate your results; then explore one, two, or more of twenty-eight faiths/spiritual paths followed in America today. "An innovative and entertaining way to think—and rethink—about your own spiritual path, or perhaps even to find one." —Dan Wakefield, author of *How Do We Know When It's God?*
6 x 9, 160 pp, Quality PB, ISBN 1-893361-08-X **$15.95**

Spiritual Manifestos: *Visions for Renewed Religious Life in America from Young Spiritual Leaders of Many Faiths*
Edited by *Niles Elliot Goldstein*; Preface by *Martin E. Marty*

Discover the reasons why so many people have kept organized religion at arm's length.

Here, ten young spiritual leaders, most in their mid-thirties, representing the spectrum of religious traditions—Protestant, Catholic, Jewish, Buddhist, Unitarian Universalist—present the innovative ways they are transforming our spiritual communities and our lives. "These ten articulate young spiritual leaders engender hope for the vitality of 21st-century religion." —Forrest Church, Minister of All Souls Church in New York City
6 x 9, 256 pp, HC, ISBN 1-893361-09-8 **$21.95**

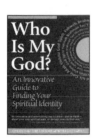 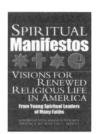 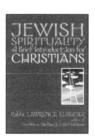 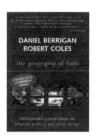

Jewish Spirituality: *A Brief Introduction for Christians*
by *Lawrence Kushner*

Lawrence Kushner, whose award-winning books have brought Jewish spirituality to life for countless readers of all faiths and backgrounds, tailors his unique style to address Christians' questions, revealing the essence of Judaism in a way that people whose own tradition traces its roots to Judaism can understand and enjoy.
5½ x 8½, 112 pp, Quality PB, ISBN 1-58023-150-0 **$12.95**

The Geography of Faith
Underground Conversations on Religious, Political and Social Change
by *Daniel Berrigan* and *Robert Coles*; Updated introduction and afterword by the authors

A classic of faith-based activism—updated for a new generation.

Listen in on the conversations between these two great teachers—one a renegade priest wanted by the FBI for his protests against the Vietnam war, the other a future Pulitzer Prize-winning journalist—as they struggle with what it means to put your faith to the test. Discover how their story of challenging the status quo during a time of great political, religious, and social change is just as applicable to our lives today. 6 x 9, 224 pp, Quality PB, ISBN 1-893361-40-3 **$16.95**

Spiritual Biography

The Life of Evelyn Underhill
An Intimate Portrait of the Ground-Breaking Author of Mysticism
by *Margaret Cropper*; Foreword by *Dana Greene*

Evelyn Underhill was a passionate writer and teacher who wrote elegantly on mysticism, worship, and devotional life. This is the story of how she made her way toward spiritual maturity, from her early days of agnosticism to the years when her influence was felt throughout the world. 6 x 9, 288 pp, 5+ b/w photos, Quality PB, ISBN 1-893361-70-5 **$18.95**

Zen Effects: *The Life of Alan Watts*
by *Monica Furlong*

The first and only full-length biography of one of the most charismatic spiritual leaders of the twentieth century—now back in print!

Through his widely popular books and lectures, Alan Watts (1915–1973) did more to introduce Eastern philosophy and religion to Western minds than any figure before or since. Here is the only biography of this charismatic figure, who served as Zen teacher, Anglican priest, lecturer, academic, entertainer, a leader of the San Francisco renaissance, and author of more than 30 books, including *The Way of Zen, Psychotherapy East and West* and *The Spirit of Zen.*
6 x 9, 264 pp, Quality PB, ISBN 1-893361-32-2 **$16.95**

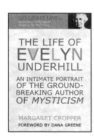 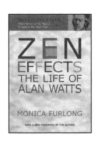 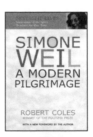 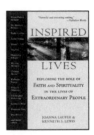

Simone Weil: *A Modern Pilgrimage*
by *Robert Coles*

The extraordinary life of the spiritual philosopher who's been called both saint and madwoman.

The French writer and philosopher Simone Weil (1906–1943) devoted her life to a search for God—while avoiding membership in organized religion. Robert Coles' intriguing study of Weil details her short, eventful life, and is an insightful portrait of the beloved and controversial thinker whose life and writings influenced many (from T. S. Eliot to Adrienne Rich to Albert Camus), and continue to inspire seekers everywhere. 6 x 9, 208 pp, Quality PB, ISBN 1-893361-34-9 **$16.95**

Inspired Lives: *Exploring the Role of Faith and Spirituality in the Lives of Extraordinary People*
by *Joanna Laufer* and *Kenneth S. Lewis*

Contributors include *Ang Lee, Wynton Marsalis, Kathleen Norris, Hakeem Olajuwon, Christopher Parkening, Madeleine L'Engle, Doc Watson,* and many more

In this moving book, soul-searching conversations unearth the importance of spirituality and personal faith for more than forty artists and innovators who have made a real difference in our world through their work. 6 x 9, 256 pp, Quality PB, ISBN 1-893361-33-0 **$16.95**

Spiritual Practice

Women Pray
Voices through the Ages, from Many Faiths, Cultures, and Traditions
Edited and with introductions by *Monica Furlong*

Many ways—new and old—to communicate with the Divine.

This beautiful gift book celebrates the rich variety of ways women around the world have called out to the Divine—with words of joy, praise, gratitude, wonder, petition, longing, and even anger—from the ancient world up to our own time. Prayers from women of nearly every religious or spiritual background give us an eloquent expression of what it means to communicate with God. 5 x7¼,256 pp, Deluxe HC with ribbon marker, ISBN 1-893361-25-X **$19.95**

Praying with Our Hands: *Twenty-One Practices of Embodied Prayer from the World's Spiritual Traditions*
by *Jon M. Sweeney*; Photographs by *Jennifer J. Wilson*;
Foreword by *Mother Tessa Bielecki*; Afterword by *Taitetsu Unno, Ph.D.*

A spiritual guidebook for bringing prayer into our bodies.

This inspiring book of reflections and accompanying photographs shows us twenty-one simple ways of using our hands to speak to God, to enrich our devotion and ritual. All express the various approaches of the world's religious traditions to bringing the body into worship. Spiritual traditions represented include Anglican, Sufi, Zen, Roman Catholic, Yoga, Shaker, Hindu, Jewish, Pentecostal, Eastern Orthodox, and many others.
8 x 8, 96 pp, 22 duotone photographs, Quality PB, ISBN 1-893361-16-0 **$16.95**

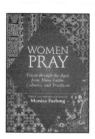 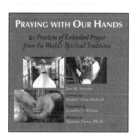 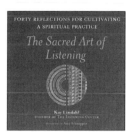 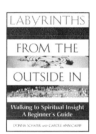

The Sacred Art of Listening
Forty Reflections for Cultivating a Spiritual Practice
by *Kay Lindahl*; Illustrations by *Amy Schnapper*

More than ever before, we need to embrace the skills and practice of listening. You will learn to: Speak clearly from your heart • Communicate with courage and compassion • Heighten your awareness for deep listening • Enhance your ability to listen to people with different belief systems. 8 x 8, 160 pp, Illus., Quality PB, ISBN 1-893361-44-6 **$16.95**

Labyrinths from the Outside In
Walking to Spiritual Insight—a Beginner's Guide
by *Donna Schaper* and *Carole Ann Camp*

The user-friendly, interfaith guide to making and using labyrinths— for meditation, prayer, and celebration.

Labyrinth walking is a spiritual exercise *anyone* can do. This accessible guide unlocks the mysteries of the labyrinth for all of us, providing ideas for using the labyrinth walk for prayer, meditation, and celebrations to mark the most important moments in life. Includes instructions for making a labyrinth of your own and finding one in your area.
6 x 9, 208 pp, b/w illus. and photographs, Quality PB, ISBN 1-893361-18-7 **$16.95**

Spirituality

One God Clapping: *The Spiritual Path of a Zen Rabbi*
by *Alan Lew* with *Sherril Jaffe*

Firsthand account of a spiritual journey from Zen Buddhist practitioner to rabbi.

A fascinating personal story of a Jewish meditation expert's roundabout spiritual journey from Zen Buddhist practitioner to rabbi. An insightful source of inspiration for each of us who is on the journey to find God in today's multi-faceted spiritual world.
5½ x 8½, 336 pp, Quality PB, ISBN 1-58023-115-2 **$16.95**

Aleph-Bet Yoga
Embodying the Hebrew Letters for Physical and Spiritual Well-Being
by *Steven A. Rapp*; Foreword by *Tamar Frankiel* & *Judy Greenfeld*; Preface by *Hart Lazer*

Blends aspects of hatha yoga and the shapes of the Hebrew letters. Connects yoga practice with Jewish spiritual life. Easy-to-follow instructions, b/w photos.
7 x 10, 128 pp, Quality PB, b/w photos, ISBN 1-58023-162-4 **$16.95**

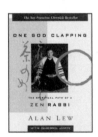 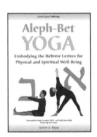 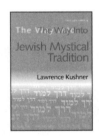 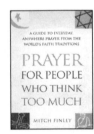

The Way Into Jewish Mystical Tradition
by *Lawrence Kushner*

Explains the principles of Jewish mystical thinking, their religious and spiritual significance, and how they relate to our lives. A book that allows us to experience and understand the Jewish mystical approach to our place in the world.
6 x 9, 224 pp, HC, ISBN 1-58023-029-6 **$21.95**

Prayer for People Who Think Too Much
A Guide to Everyday, Anywhere Prayer from the World's Faith Traditions
by *Mitch Finley*

Helps us make prayer a natural part of daily living.

Takes a thoughtful look at how each major faith tradition incorporates prayer into *daily* life. Explores Christian sacraments, Jewish holy days, Muslim daily prayer, "mindfulness" in Buddhism, and more, to help you better understand and enhance your own prayer practices.
"I love this book." —Caroline Myss, author of *Anatomy of the Spirit*
5½ x 8½, 224 pp, Quality PB, ISBN 1-893361-21-7 **$16.95**; HC, ISBN 1-893361-00-4 **$21.95**

SkyLight Illuminations Series
Andrew Harvey, series editor

Offers today's spiritual seeker an enjoyable entry into the great classic texts of the world's spiritual traditions. Each classic is presented in an accessible translation, with facing pages of guided commentary from experts, giving you the keys you need to understand the history, context, and meaning of the text. This series enables readers of all backgrounds to experience and understand classic spiritual texts directly, and to make them a part of their lives. Andrew Harvey writes the foreword to each volume, an insightful, personal introduction to each classic.

Bhagavad Gita: *Annotated & Explained*
Translation by *Shri Purohit Swami*; Annotation by *Kendra Crossen Burroughs*

"The very best Gita for first-time readers." —Ken Wilber

Millions of people turn daily to India's most beloved holy book, whose universal appeal has made it popular with non-Hindus and Hindus alike. This edition introduces you to the characters; explains references and philosophical terms; shares the interpretations of famous spiritual leaders and scholars; and more. 5½ x 8½, 192 pp, Quality PB, ISBN 1-893361-28-4 **$15.95**

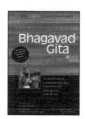 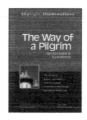 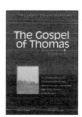

The Way of a Pilgrim: *Annotated & Explained*
Translation and annotation by *Gleb Pokrovsky*

The classic of Russian spirituality—now with facing-page commentary that illuminates and explains the text for you.

This delightful account is the story of one man who sets out to learn the prayer of the heart— also known as the "Jesus prayer"—and how the practice transforms his existence. This edition guides you through an abridged version of the text with facing-page annotations explaining the names, terms and references. 5½ x 8½, 160 pp, Quality PB, ISBN 1-893361-31-4 **$14.95**

The Gospel of Thomas: *Annotated & Explained*
Translation and annotation by *Stevan Davies*

The recently discovered mystical sayings of Jesus—now with facing-page commentary that illuminates and explains the text for you.

Discovered in 1945, this collection of aphoristic sayings sheds new light on the origins of Christianity and the intriguing figure of Jesus, portraying the Kingdom of God as a present fact about the world, rather than a future promise or future threat. This edition guides you through the text with annotations that focus on the meaning of the sayings, ideal for readers with no previous background in Christian history or thought. 5½ x 8½, 192 pp, Quality PB, ISBN 1-893361-45-4 **$15.95**

SkyLight Illuminations Series
Andrew Harvey, series editor

Zohar: *Annotated & Explained*
Translation and annotation by *Daniel C. Matt*

The cornerstone text of Kabbalah, now with facing-page commentary that illuminates and explains the text for you.

The best-selling author of *The Essential Kabbalah* brings together in one place the most important teachings of the *Zohar*, the canonical text of Jewish mystical tradition. Guides readers step by step through the midrash, mystical fantasy and Hebrew scripture that make up the *Zohar*, explaining the inner meanings in facing-page commentary. Ideal for readers without any prior knowledge of Jewish mysticism.

5½ x 8½, 176 pp, Quality PB, ISBN 1-893361-51-9 **$15.95**

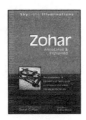 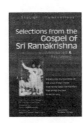 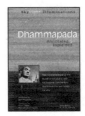

Selections from the Gospel of Sri Ramakrishna
Annotated & Explained
Translation by *Swami Nikhilananda*; Annotation by *Kendra Crossen Burroughs*

The words of India's greatest example of God-consciousness and mystical ecstasy in recent history—now with facing-page commentary that illuminates and explains the text for you.

Introduces the fascinating world of the Indian mystic and the universal appeal of his message that has inspired millions of devotees for more than a century. Selections from the original text and insightful yet unobtrusive commentary highlight the most important and inspirational teachings. Ideal for readers without any prior knowledge of Hinduism.

5½ x 8½, 240 pp, b/w photographs, Quality PB, ISBN 1-893361-46-2 **$16.95**

Dhammapada: *Annotated & Explained*
Translation by *Max Müller*; Annotation by *Jack Maguire*

The classic of Buddhist spiritual practice—now with facing-page commentary that illuminates and explains the text for you.

The Dhammapada—words spoken by the Buddha himself over 2,500 years ago—is notoriously difficult to understand for the first-time reader. Now you can experience it with understanding even if you have no previous knowledge of Buddhism. Enlightening facing-page commentary explains all the names, terms, and references, giving you deeper insight into the text. An excellent introduction to Buddhist life and practice.

5½ x 8½, 160 pp, Quality PB, ISBN 1-893361-42-X **$14.95**

Meditation/Prayer

Finding Grace at the Center: *The Beginning of Centering Prayer*

by *M. Basil Pennington, OCSO, Thomas Keating, OCSO,* and *Thomas E. Clarke, SJ*

The book that helped launch the Centering Prayer "movement." Explains the prayer of *The Cloud of Unknowing,* posture and relaxation, the three simple rules of centering prayer, and how to cultivate centering prayer throughout all aspects of your life.
5 x 7¼, 112 pp, HC, ISBN 1-893361-69-1 **$14.95**

Three Gates to Meditation Practice
A Personal Journey into Sufism, Buddhism, and Judaism
by *David A. Cooper*

Shows us how practicing within more than one spiritual tradition can lead us to our true home.

Here are over fifteen years from the journey of "post-denominational rabbi" David A. Cooper, author of *God Is a Verb,* and his wife, Shoshana—years in which the Coopers explored a rich variety of practices, from chanting Sufi *dhikr* to Buddhist Vipassanā meditation, to the study of Kabbalah and esoteric Judaism. Their experience demonstrates that the spiritual path is really completely within our reach, whoever we are, whatever we do—as long as we are willing to practice it. 5½ x 8½, 240 pp, Quality PB, ISBN 1-893361-22-5 **$16.95**

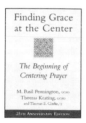 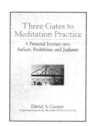 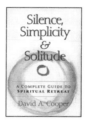 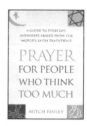

Silence, Simplicity & Solitude
A Complete Guide to Spiritual Retreat at Home
by *David A. Cooper*

The classic personal spiritual retreat guide that enables readers to create their own self-guided spiritual retreat at home.

Award-winning author David Cooper traces personal mystical retreat in all of the world's major traditions, describing the varieties of spiritual practices for modern spiritual seekers. Cooper shares the techniques and practices that encompass the personal spiritual retreat experience, allowing readers to enhance their meditation practices and create an effective, self-guided spiritual retreat in their own homes—without the instruction of a meditation teacher. 5½ x 8½, 336 pp, Quality PB, ISBN 1-893361-04-7 **$16.95**

Prayer for People Who Think Too Much
A Guide to Everyday, Anywhere Prayer from the World's Faith Traditions
by *Mitch Finley*

Helps us make prayer a natural part of daily living.

Takes a thoughtful look at how each major faith tradition incorporates prayer into *daily* life. Explores Christian sacraments, Jewish holy days, Muslim daily prayer, "mindfulness" in Buddhism, and more, to help you better understand and enhance your own prayer practices. "I love this book." —Caroline Myss, author of *Anatomy of the Spirit*
5½ x 8½, 224 pp, Quality PB, ISBN 1-893361-21-7 **$16.95**; HC, ISBN 1-893361-00-4 **$21.95**

Kabbalah

Honey from the Rock
An Introduction to Jewish Mysticism
by *Lawrence Kushner*

An insightful and absorbing introduction to the ten gates of Jewish mysticism and how it applies to daily life. "The easiest introduction to Jewish mysticism you can read."
6 x 9, 176 pp, Quality PB, ISBN 1-58023-073-3 **$15.95**

Eyes Remade for Wonder
The Way of Jewish Mysticism and Sacred Living
A Lawrence Kushner Reader
Intro. by *Thomas Moore*, author of *Care of the Soul*

Whether you are new to Kushner or a devoted fan, you'll find inspiration here. With samplings from each of Kushner's works, and a generous amount of new material, this book is to be read and reread, each time discovering deeper layers of meaning in our lives.
6 x 9, 240 pp, Quality PB, ISBN 1-58023-042-3 **$16.95**; HC, ISBN 1-58023-014-8 **$23.95**

Invisible Lines of Connection
Sacred Stories of the Ordinary
by *Lawrence Kushner* AWARD WINNER!

Through his everyday encounters with family, friends, colleagues and strangers, Kushner takes us deeply into our lives, finding flashes of spiritual insight in the process.
5½ x 8½, 160 pp, Quality PB, ISBN 1-879045-98-2 **$15.95**

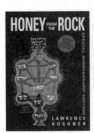 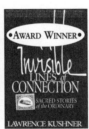 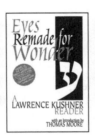 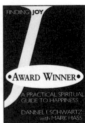 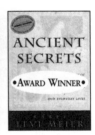

Finding Joy
A Practical Spiritual Guide to Happiness
by *Dannel I. Schwartz* with *Mark Hass* AWARD WINNER!

Explains how to find joy through a time honored, creative—and surprisingly practical—approach based on the teachings of Jewish mysticism and Kabbalah.
6 x 9, 192 pp, Quality PB, ISBN 1-58023-009-1 **$14.95**; HC, ISBN 1-879045-53-2 **$19.95**

Ancient Secrets
Using the Stories of the Bible to Improve Our Everyday Lives
by *Rabbi Levi Meier, Ph.D.* AWARD WINNER!

Drawing on a broad range of wisdom writings, distinguished rabbi and psychologist Levi Meier takes a thoughtful, wise and fresh approach to showing us how to apply the stories of the Bible to our everyday lives.
5½ x 8½, 288 pp, Quality PB, ISBN 1-58023-064-4 **$16.95**

Children's Spirituality

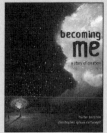

Becoming Me: *A Story of Creation*
by *Martin Boroson*
Full-color illus. by *Christopher Gilvan-Cartwright*

For ages 4 & up

Told in the personal "voice" of the Creator, here is a story about creation and relationship that is about each one of us. In simple words and with radiant illustrations, the Creator tells an intimate story about love, about friendship and playing, about our world—and about ourselves. And with each turn of the page, we're reminded that we just might be closer to our Creator than we think!

8 x 10, 32 pp, Full-color illus., HC, ISBN 1-893361-11-X **$16.95**

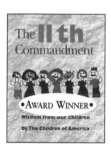 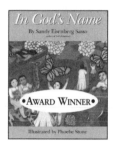 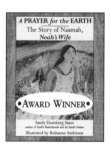

A Prayer for the Earth
The Story of Naamah, Noah's Wife
by *Sandy Eisenberg Sasso*
Full-color illus. by *Bethanne Andersen*

For ages 4 & up

This new story, based on an ancient text, opens readers' religious imaginations to new ideas about the well-known story of the Flood. When God tells Noah to bring the animals of the world onto the ark, God also calls on Naamah, Noah's wife, to save each plant on Earth. "A lovely tale.... Children of all ages should be drawn to this parable for our times." —Tomie de Paola, artist/author of books for children
9 x 12, 32 pp, HC, Full-color illus., ISBN 1-879045-60-5 **$16.95**

In God's Name

For ages 4 & up

by *Sandy Eisenberg Sasso*; Full-color illus. by *Phoebe Stone*

Like an ancient myth in its poetic text and vibrant illustrations, this award-winning modern fable about the search for God's name celebrates the diversity and, at the same time, the unity of all the people of the world.
9 x 12, 32 pp, HC, Full-color illus., ISBN 1-879045-26-5 **$16.95**

Also available in Spanish:
El nombre de Dios 9 x 12, 32 pp, HC, Full-color illus., ISBN 1-893361-63-2 **$16.95**

The 11th Commandment
Wisdom from Our Children
by *The Children of America*

For ages 4 & up

"If there were an Eleventh Commandment, what would it be?" Children of many religious denominations across America answer this question—in their own drawings and words. "A rare book of spiritual celebration for all people, of all ages, for all time." —*Bookviews*
8 x 10, 48 pp, HC, Full-color illus., ISBN 1-879045-46-X **$16.95**

Children's Spirituality

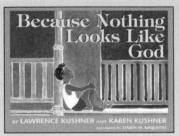

Because Nothing Looks Like God
by *Lawrence and Karen Kushner*
Full-color illus. by
Dawn W. Majewski

For ages 4 & up

MULTICULTURAL, NONDENOMINATIONAL,
NONSECTARIAN

Real-life examples of happiness and sadness—from goodnight stories, to the hope and fear felt the first time at bat, to the closing moments of life—introduce children to the possibilities of spiritual life. A vibrant way for children—and their adults—to explore what, where, and how God is in our lives.

11 x 8½, 32 pp, HC, Full-color illus., ISBN 1-58023-092-X **$16.95**

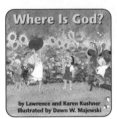
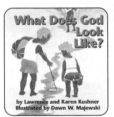
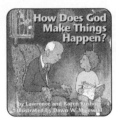
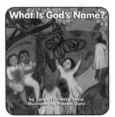

Where Is God? (A Board Book)
by *Lawrence and Karen Kushner*; Full-color illus. by *Dawn W. Majewski*

For ages 0–4

A gentle way for young children to explore how God is with us every day, in every way. Abridged from *Because Nothing Looks Like God* by Lawrence and Karen Kushner and specially adapted to board book format to delight and inspire young readers.
5 x 5, 24 pp, Board, Full-color illus., ISBN 1-893361-17-9 **$7.95**

What Does God Look Like? (A Board Book)
by *Lawrence and Karen Kushner*; Full-color illus. by *Dawn W. Majewski*

For ages 0–4

A simple way for young children to explore the ways that we "see" God. Abridged from *Because Nothing Looks Like God* by Lawrence and Karen Kushner and specially adapted to board book format to delight and inspire young readers.
5 x 5, 24 pp, Board, Full-color illus., ISBN 1-893361-23-3 **$7.95**

How Does God Make Things Happen? (A Board Book)
by *Lawrence and Karen Kushner*; Full-color illus. by *Dawn W. Majewski*

For ages 0–4

A charming invitation for young children to explore how God makes things happen in our world. Abridged from *Because Nothing Looks Like God* by Lawrence and Karen Kushner and specially adapted to board book format to delight and inspire young readers.
5 x 5, 24 pp, Board, Full-color illus., ISBN 1-893361-24-1 **$7.95**

What Is God's Name? (A Board Book)
by *Sandy Eisenberg Sasso*; Full-color illus. by *Phoebe Stone*

For ages 0–4

Everyone and everything in the world has a name. What is God's name? Abridged from the award-winning *In God's Name* by Sandy Eisenberg Sasso and specially adapted to board book format to delight and inspire young readers.
5 x 5, 24 pp, Board, Full-color illus., ISBN 1-893361-10-1 **$7.95**

Children's Spirituality

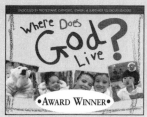

Where Does God Live?

For ages 3–6

by *August Gold* and *Matthew J. Perlman*

Using simple, everyday examples that children can relate to, this colorful book helps young readers develop a personal understanding of God.

10 x 8½, 32 pp, Quality PB, Full-color photo illus.,
ISBN 1-893361-39-X **$7.95**

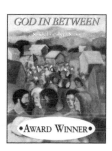

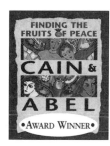

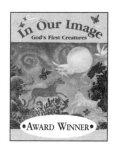

God in Between

For ages 4 & up

by *Sandy Eisenberg Sasso*; Full-color illus. by *Sally Sweetland*

If you wanted to find God, where would you look? A magical, mythical tale that teaches that God can be found where we are: within all of us and the relationships between us. "This happy and wondrous book takes our children on a sweet and holy journey into God's presence." —Rabbi Wayne Dosick, Ph.D., author of *The Business Bible* and *Soul Judaism*
9 x 12, 32 pp, HC, Full-color illus., ISBN 1-879045-86-9 **$16.95**

Cain & Abel: *Finding the Fruits of Peace*

For ages 5 & up

by *Sandy Eisenberg Sasso*; Full-color illus. by *Joani Keller Rothenberg*

A sensitive recasting of the ancient tale shows we have the power to deal with anger in positive ways. Provides questions for kids and adults to explore together. "Editor's Choice"—American Library Association's *Booklist*
9 x 12, 32 pp, HC, Full-color illus., ISBN 1-58023-123-3 **$16.95**

In Our Image: *God's First Creatures*

For ages 4 & up

by *Nancy Sohn Swartz*; Full-color illus. by *Melanie Hall*

A playful new twist on the Creation story—from the perspective of the animals. Celebrates the interconnectedness of nature and the harmony of all living things. "The vibrantly colored illustrations nearly leap off the page in this delightful interpretation." —*School Library Journal*
"A message all children should hear, presented in words and pictures that children will find irresistible." —Rabbi Harold Kushner, author of *When Bad Things Happen to Good People*
9 x 12, 32 pp, HC, Full-color illus., ISBN 1-879045-99-0 **$16.95**

Children's Spirituality

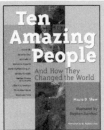

Ten Amazing People
And How They Changed the World
by *Maura D. Shaw*; Foreword by *Dr. Robert Coles*
Full-color illus. by *Stephen Marchesi*

For ages 6–10

Black Elk • Dorothy Day • Malcolm X • Mahatma Gandhi • Martin Luther King, Jr. • Mother Teresa • Janusz Korczak • Desmond Tutu • Thich Nhat Hanh • Albert Schweitzer

This vivid, inspirational, and authoritative book will open new possibilities for children by telling the stories of how ten of the past century's greatest leaders changed the world in important ways.

8½, x 11, 48 pp, HC, Full-color illus., ISBN 1-893361-47-0 **$17.95**

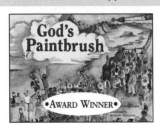

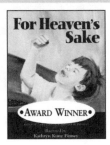

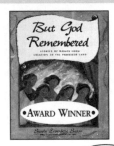

God's Paintbrush

For ages 4 & up

by *Sandy Eisenberg Sasso*; Full-color illus. by *Annette Compton*

Invites children of all faiths and backgrounds to encounter God openly in their own lives. Wonderfully interactive; provides questions adult and child can explore together at the end of each episode. "An excellent way to honor the imaginative breadth and depth of the spiritual life of the young." —Dr. Robert Coles, Harvard University
11 x 8½, 32 pp, HC, Full-color illus., ISBN 1-879045-22-2 **$16.95**

Also available:
A Teacher's Guide 8½ x 11, 32 pp, PB, ISBN 1-879045-57-5 **$8.95**
God's Paintbrush Celebration Kit 9½ x 12, HC, Includes 5 sessions/40 full-color Activity Sheets and Teacher Folder with complete instructions, ISBN 1-58023-050-4 **$21.95**

For Heaven's Sake

For ages 4 & up

by *Sandy Eisenberg Sasso*; Full-color illus. by *Kathryn Kunz Finney*

Everyone talked about heaven, but no one would say what heaven was or how to find it. So Isaiah decides to find out, by seeking answers from many different people. "This book is a reminder of how well Sandy Sasso knows the minds of children. But it may surprise—and delight—readers to find how well she knows us grown-ups too." —Maria Harris, National Consultant in Religious Education, and author of *Teaching and Religious Imagination*
9 x 12, 32 pp, HC, Full-color illus., ISBN 1-58023-054-7 **$16.95**

But God Remembered
Stories of Women from Creation to the Promised Land

For ages 8 & up

by *Sandy Eisenberg Sasso*; Full-color illus. by *Bethanne Andersen*

Vibrantly brings to life four stories of courageous and strong women from ancient tradition; all teach important values through their actions and faith. "Exquisite.... A book of beauty, strength and spirituality." —Association of Bible Teachers
9 x 12, 32 pp, HC, Full-color illus., ISBN 1-879045-43-5 **$16.95**

Religious Etiquette/Reference

How to Be a Perfect Stranger, In 2 Volumes
A Guide to Etiquette in Other People's Religious Ceremonies
Ed. by *Stuart M. Matlins* and *Arthur J. Magida* **AWARD WINNERS!**

Explains the rituals and celebrations of North America's major religions/denominations, helping an interested guest to feel comfortable, participate to the fullest extent possible, and avoid violating anyone's religious principles. Answers practical questions from the perspective of *any* other faith.

Vol. 1: North America's Largest Faiths
VOL. 1 COVERS: Assemblies of God • Baptist • Buddhist • Christian Church (Disciples of Christ) • Christian Science • Churches of Christ • Episcopalian/Anglican • Greek Orthodox • Hindu • Islam • Jehovah's Witnesses • Jewish • Lutheran • Methodist • Mormon • Presbyterian • Quaker • Roman Catholic • Seventh-day Adventist • United Church of Canada • United Church of Christ 6 x 9, 432 pp, Quality PB, ISBN 1-893361-01-2 **$19.95**

Vol. 2: More Faiths in North America
VOL. 2 COVERS: African American Methodist Churches • Baha'i • Christian and Missionary Alliance • Christian Congregation • Church of the Brethren • Church of the Nazarene • Evangelical Free Church • International Church of the Foursquare Gospel • International Pentecostal Holiness Church • Mennonite/Amish • Native American/First Nations • Orthodox Churches • Pentecostal Church of God • Reformed Church • Sikh • Unitarian Universalist • Wesleyan 6 x 9, 416 pp, Quality PB, ISBN 1-893361-02-0 **$19.95**

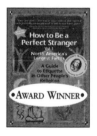 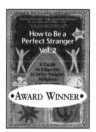 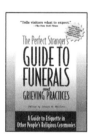 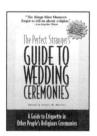

Also available:

The Perfect Stranger's Guide to Funerals and Grieving Practices
A Guide to Etiquette in Other People's Religious Ceremonies
Edited by *Stuart M. Matlins*
6 x 9, 240 pp, Quality PB, ISBN 1-893361-20-9 **$16.95**

The Perfect Stranger's Guide to Wedding Ceremonies
A Guide to Etiquette in Other People's Religious Ceremonies
Edited by *Stuart M. Matlins*
6 x 9, 208 pp, Quality PB, ISBN 1-893361-19-5 **$16.95**

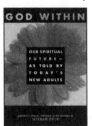 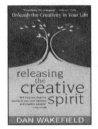 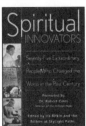